SAYING GOODBYE IN CHILD PSYCHOTHERAPY

CHILD THERAPY SERIES

A Series of Books Edited By

Charles Schaefer

SAYING GOODBYE IN CHILD PSYCHOTHERAPY

Planned, Unplanned, and Premature Endings

DONNA CANGELOSI, PSY.D.

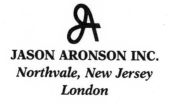

JASON ARONSON INC.
Northvale, New Jersey
London

Production Editor: Elaine Lindenblatt

This book was set in 11 pt. New Aster by Alabama Book Composition of Deatsville, Alabama, and printed and bound by Book-mart Press, Inc. of North Bergen, New Jersey.

Library of Congress Cataloging-in-Publication Data

Cangelosi, Donna M.
    Saying goodbye in child psychotherapy : planned, unplanned, and premature endings / Donna Cangelosi.
      p. cm.
    Includes bibliographical references and index.
    ISBN 1-56821-677-7 (alk. paper)
    1. Child psychotherapy—Termination. 2. Play therapy. I. Title.
RJ505.T47C36   1997
618.92′8914—dc21   96-49473

Printed in the United States of America on acid-free paper. For information and catalog write to Jason Aronson Inc., 230 Livingston Street, Northvale, New Jersey 07647-1731. Or visit our website: http://www.aronson.com

To Scott

CONTENTS

Part Two: Planned Endings
Following Successful Treatment

Part Three: Premature Endings

PREFACE

"In every ending lies the potential for a new beginning." These words or some variation on them were expressed to me on a regular basis during the late spring and early summer of 1994. It was at that time that I was offered a university position requiring that I relocate and leave my practice. Among the many challenges that confronted me was the task of saying goodbye to my patients, in the midst of their treatment, before a "natural" ending would be possible. This resulted in a wide variety of personal reactions ranging from satisfaction and accomplishment to sadness, guilt, and a sense of loss and mourning.

I was aware that there was no one model for ending treatment that could address the specific needs and issues of all of my patients. Furthermore, I was unable to locate an "expert" or a book that specifically focused on terminating treatment with children of various ages and diagnostic groups. This experience propelled me to read as much as possible about mourning and the termination process. Some of the most poignant moments during this period took place in my play room, where dramatic and immensely creative expressions of mourning, letting go, holding on, abandonment, killing off, dying, and rebirth were played out. *Saying Goodbye in Child Psychotherapy* is a synthesis of research, personal experience, and professional insights. It was inspired by the reactions of children when I moved and during other planned and premature terminations. I have repeatedly been struck by the unique ways in which children have let go of treatment and the powerful ways they have used play to do so.

I have noticed that in the education of child psychotherapists little attention is paid to dealing with termination. In child therapy classes and workshops, colleagues as well as students frequently ask questions about the ideal time for ending treatment. This issue becomes rather confusing when, in spite of therapeutic progress, a child's family remains chaotic or unsupportive or the child is approaching a difficult developmental phase (e.g., preadolescence).

Saying Goodbye in Child Psychotherapy is intended as an aid for students and practitioners of child therapy and counseling, including psychologists, social workers, psychiatrists, psychiatric nurses, and candidates in analytic institutes. It is best used as a supplement to coursework and professional supervision. The book is designed as a manual that will guide child clinicians through a variety of different kinds of terminations. Through both theoretical information and clinical case material, *Saying Goodbye in Child Psychotherapy* shows how child therapists can tailor play and art techniques and materials to specific situations, discusses emotional issues that come up for both child and therapist, and illustrates effective ways of handling emotional reactions and the termination process in general.

ACKNOWLEDGMENTS

An eight-year-old boy created a poignant separation scene with felt animals when we discussed ending treatment. This child's creative use of play inspired me to write a fifteen-page case study in which the ending phase of child psychotherapy was addressed. The original case study (in Chapter 8) later evolved into a book proposal, thanks to the encouragement of Dr. Charles Schaefer. It was his enthusiasm about the topic that motivated me to take on the task of writing a book.

I wish to thank Dr. Jason Aronson for his confidence in my writing ability and for sharing his vision for this book. I am also grateful to Norma Pomerantz, Dr. Michael Moskowitz, and Elaine Lindenblatt at Aronson Publishers who enthusiastically and consistently took the time to help me with the many small details this project entailed. Special thanks also to Dr. Tamara Shulman who contributed her knowledge and experience regarding children's reactions to the pregnancy of a therapist, and to Cheryl Nifoussi, M.S.W., for critiquing the manuscript and sharing her expertise in psychoanalytic theory.

The support and encouragement of my dear friends Aurora, Billy, and Dr. Joe Braun also contributed to the completion of this project. Finally and most of all, I wish to acknowledge my husband and best friend, Scott James, who encouraged me to write this book; helped me with research, editing, and printing details; and contributed his artistic talent to the Appendix.

INTRODUCTION

For the child to start analysis is a step toward permitting him to break away from mother. An analyst who respects the child's autonomy will, as a new object, foster separation from adults. Through identification with the analyst, the child will often learn adaptive means of independence.

Jules Glenn

Most clinicians would agree that the termination phase of treatment is both important and, at times, difficult to deal with. Despite the fact that termination is an inevitable phase of all treatment, it has been addressed less frequently in the psychoanalytic literature than other aspects of analysis (e.g. the initial phase of treatment and issues related to technique, transference, countertransference, and resistance). The topic of termination is dealt with even less in literature dealing with psychotherapy. This is especially true in the area of child psychotherapy.

It has been argued (Levinson 1977, Mozgal 1985) that the relatively limited amount of literature on the topic of termination is a result of clinicians distancing themselves from issues related to separation and letting go. A review of the literature indicates that most authors who do discuss the topic of terminating child psychotherapy do so without significant detail and with minimal focus on the emotions of either child or therapist. Most of the more indepth work about termination issues with children has been introduced by child analysts (Gillman 1991).

In contrast to child analysts, psychotherapists often pay little attention to the meaning of termination for child patients. It is frequently assumed that children will not be affected by ending treatment because of the presence, stability, and/or sensitivity of their parents (or other supports). This line of thinking can serve to cushion emotions related to ending treatment for both the child and the therapist and, in some cases, can cause the therapist to minimize his or her unique role in the child's life. On the opposite side of the coin, when treating children from chaotic, abusive, and/or resistant families, therapists may come to feel helpless regarding the impact that treatment can have. This is often indicative of a countertransferential reaction, but in either case such feelings can cause the therapist to deny the important roles that psychotherapy and the therapeutic relationship serve for the child.

Gillman (1991) notes that it is often assumed that, because psychotherapy takes place less frequently and often over a shorter span of time, it does not bring about as strong an attachment as does psychoanalysis. He believes that "childism" prevents many therapists from seeing the importance of the termination with children. Gillman defines childism as "a tendency to avoid the enormous significance of the therapist to the child" and attributes it to "ignorance, countertransference, and the child's relative inability to verbalize his feelings" (p. 340).

Regardless of the reason(s) why child psychotherapists do not focus on termination issues, minimizing their importance to the child can convey the message that what the child feels or thinks about saying goodbye is not important or okay to talk about. Most children will have some reaction to the impending separation and will tend to interpret its meaning on the basis of their age, cognitive ability, ethnic and cultural background, temperament, and previous experience with separation, loss, or abandonment. The manner in which the therapist addresses termination issues will give the child a message, good or bad, about how to deal with feelings related to a significant ending.

Gillman (1991) notes that even once-a-week therapy lasting for just a few weeks requires an awareness and sensitivity to issues that may emerge in ending treatment. When preparing for termination, children need the assistance of their therapist to address issues related to attachment, separation, loss, mourning, emancipation, and whatever other feelings are elicited by this significant ending. Play and art therapies allow the clinician to provide this assistance in a manner that is sensitive to the child's developmental needs. They allow the child's thoughts and feelings to emerge in a disguised form that provides a sense of psychological safety. These therapeutic properties are particularly important during the termination phase of treatment, as it is during this period that uncomfortable feelings about the therapist often emerge. It is not uncommon for children to feel anger or even rage toward the therapist, for therapists to be viewed with jealousy or envy, or for children to feel elated, joyful, or free as a result of terminating treatment. In each instance, children are unable to express such strong and often confusing emotions directly. Play and art therapies provide the child with an opportunity to work through these feelings in a comfortable, non-threatening manner.

This book is organized in four major sections:

Part One: *Theoretical Background* explores psychoanalytic and developmental principles for determining the timing and appropriateness of terminating treatment with children. Chapter 1 provides a framework regarding the significance of the termination phase of treatment. Two major, albeit opposing, psychoanalytic theories, that of Anna Freud and that of Frederick Allen, are discussed. Chapter 2 explores a wide range of criteria for assessing progress and readiness for termination. Developmental issues as well as mourning reactions, transference, and countertransference are explored. The use of Anna Freud's Developmental Profile as a tool for assessing readiness for termination is then described in Chapter 3.

Part Two: *Planned Endings Following Successful Treatment* explores the importance of chronological age and developmental challenges during the ending phase of treatment. Chapters 4 and 5 examine two distinct age groups: children between 3 and 5, and children between 6 and 10. Characteristics and developmental challenges, ways in which the therapist can tailor play and art therapy techniques and materials to meet developmental needs, and clinical case examples are described for each group.

Part Three: *Premature Endings* looks at terminations of treatment with children that are initiated not by clinical readiness but by changes in the child's life circumstance, parent resistance, and/or child resistance. Likewise, countertransference or changes in the therapist's life circumstance—such as relocation, illness, job change, or pregnancy—that can instigate a premature termination are explored. Chapters 6 through 8 examine these issues.

Appendix: *Structured Techniques for Saying Goodbye* provides a variety of activities that can be used with children during both planned and premature endings. This list is by no means exhaustive and I would welcome your ideas for additional techniques.

Donna Cangelosi
786 Grange Road
Teaneck, NJ 07666

PART ONE

THEORETICAL BACKGROUND

The leaving of the old and the beginning of the new constitute the ever-recurring shifting of the scenes in human development.

Frederick Allen

1

PSYCHOANALYTIC PRINCIPLES

As for our losses and gains, we have seen how often they are inextricably mixed. There is plenty we have to give up in order to grow. For we cannot deeply love anything without becoming vulnerable to loss. And we cannot become separate people, responsible people, connected people, reflective people without some losing and leaving and letting go.

Judith Viorst

Most of the literature dealing with termination has been introduced by psychoanalysts. Psychoanalytic principles regarding the ending of treatment serve as an excellent model for ending child psychotherapy. The accumulated body of knowledge that exists in this field as a result of clinical and observational research highlights the point that issues of separation and attachment are of particular developmental significance for children (Bowlby 1973, Mahler et al. 1975, Winnicott 1963). In general, the termination phase of treatment is seen as an opportunity to help children process and make connections regarding past separations and losses and to prepare for future ones. Furthermore, termination with a therapist who is close yet objective is seen as a process that can help child patients work through issues of separation and individuation.

Sigmund Freud (1937), in his paper entitled "Psychoanalysis Terminable and Interminable," was among the first clinicians to point out the importance of setting a date for the conclusion of treatment, provided that this was done "at the right time" (p. 236). He noted that termination of analysis with adults is appropriate when the patient's symptoms have dissipated and when repressed material has been dealt with so that the repetition of problems is unlikely.

The importance of simultaneously serving as a transference object and a real object for child patients makes the issue of termination a rather complex one for child analysts. While some child analysts follow the adult model for terminating treatment (i.e., setting a specific date), others see termination as only a partial separation from the child. In view of the fact that the child's development is incomplete when treatment is finished, advocates of the latter model stop treatment but do not end the therapeutic relationship. They maintain contact by planning followup sessions to see the child and/or the parents. Anna Freud argued that the child, not the therapist, determines how treatment is to progress. With regard to termination, she wrote:

> It never seemed quite logical to me that terminating a child analysis should involve the complete separation from the analyst that it usually does for adult patients. With children there is the loss of a real object as well as the loss of the transference object, and this complicates matters. To make an absolute break from a

certain date onward merely sets up another separation, and an unnecessary one. If normal progress is achieved, the child will detach himself anyway, in the course of time, just as children outgrow their nursery school teachers, their school teachers, and their friends at certain stages. The analyst can allow this detaching process to occur by reducing the frequency of visits, and often this is suggested by the child. The analyst then becomes a benign figure in the background for the child. The analyst can therafter be visited and remembered on certain occasions, and should be available for this kind of contact. [Sandler et al. 1980, p. 243]

For Anna Freud, development is a process that dictates the needs of the child at any particular point in treatment. She believed that there are clearly times when children may need to return for treatment, and thus it is important not to sever the tie to the therapist.

In contrast to Anna Freud's perspective, child analysts who adhere to the adult model of termination see it as a necessary and more or less final stage of treatment that takes place when the child's psychological and behavioral difficulties have dissipated. According to this viewpoint, a period of termination is needed so that the child can experience the problems, anxieties, and mixed emotions evoked by setting an ending date. A period of termination gives the child an opportunity to work though transference issues as well as feelings related to mourning the loss of the therapist. Advocates of this paradigm believe that not providing the child with a period in which to say goodbye leaves treatment incomplete and can result in the child's adapting a defensive resolution (Gillman 1991).

One perspective that stresses setting a date for termination has evolved from the work of Otto Rank (1929/1952). Rank believed that separation is a core, universal issue stemming from the painful experience (trauma) of birth. This experience creates a "primal anxiety" in every infant and brings about a universal desire to forget the pain, a process Rank called "primal repression." When efforts at repression are ineffective, the child develops an urge to return to the security of the womb. The struggle between the child's need to be independent and his/her simultaneous desire to return to the womb comes to a peak at certain critical periods of change and transition. Rank believed that when one "loses a closely connected person of either sex, this loss reminds one again of the primal separation from the mother. The painful task of disengaging the libido from this person (recognized by Freud in the process of mourning) corresponds to a psychical repetition of the primal trauma" (p. 25). Termination of therapy would certainly constitute such a separation according to this theory.

Frederick Allen (1942) expanded Rank's ideas and focused on issues pertaining to separation and individuation in his clinical work with children. Allen emphasized the ending phase of therapy, believing it to be one of the most important aspects of child psychotherapy: "The values of the therapeutic experience in which a child and therapist are engaged emerge in part around the fact that this relationship is begun with the goal of its eventual termination. From the first hour this is the basic orientation of the therapist" (p. 265).

Allen argued that it is important for the therapist to

help the child be an active participant in developing a plan for ending treatment. The plan for ending "becomes a positive affirmation of the child's readiness to affirm the new in himself" (p. 270). Sessions that follow the development of the plan for ending treatment provide an opportunity to address issues, anxieties, and fears related to separation. Allen proposed that the ending process carries a very strong message to the child.

> "The therapist knows that his relation to a patient is an important episode in that person's life, but that it is not, nor should it be, all of the patient's life. Thus the therapist's major interest from the beginning must be in helping the patient eventually to finish with this particular episode in his life. Only in that way can this unique relationship have any value. If a therapist adopts a protective role by trying to become a parent substitute in order to make sure before he 'lets him go' that the patient will have no further difficulties, he cannot help the child to end. No therapeutic experience can provide a patient with a paid-up insurance policy against future difficulties although the anxiety centering about ending may activate the patient's need to have such assurance. This may be and frequently is a natural part of the ending process. The therapist can meet it, however, in a way that allows it to be a part and not the whole it becomes where the orientation is focused only on the anxiety. [p. 273]

Like Anna Freud, Allen believed that there are times when children may need to return for treatment. However, he also believed that it is the very experience

of ending treatment and saying goodbye to the therapist that instills a sense of ending as a process. When
ending is seen as a process, according to Allen, it no
longer implies finality for the child. Thus the experience of ending gives children a freedom to return that
they would not otherwise have.

More often than not, termination of child treatment is initiated by outside forces such as summer
camp, the start of a new school year, moving, and the
like. Weiss (1991) stresses that children therefore need
the opportunity to disengage from treatment in whatever manner works for them. Like Weiss, I have
noticed that some children can say goodbye while
others may need to use the therapeutic relationship to
act out or even avoid issues related to ending. For
instance, children with histories of significant loss or
separation may need to set up the ending so that they
are in charge or may even attempt to abandon the
therapist by refusing to return to say goodbye. The
therapist is called upon to provide these youngsters
with a "new" way of separating, characterized by
active involvement rather than passivity or blatant
abandonment. Developmental issues also come into
play when ending treatment. Latency-age children, for
example, often distance themselves from the loss in
order to shore up their defenses. This is age appropriate and quite adaptive, especially when the decision to
stop treatment is made by someone other than the
child. The task of the therapist during termination, as
throughout treatment, is to support the child's ego in
adapting to the situation. This allows the child to leave

treatment with a sense of strength and a feeling of being supported and respected. It also plants a seed regarding the value of psychotherapy, which may foster a return to treatment at a later date.

2

CRITERIA FOR ENDING TREATMENT WITH CHILDREN

The buzzer rang. Dibs' mother was here to meet him. "Goodbye, Dibs," I said. "It's been so very nice to know you." "Yes, it has been," Dibs replied. "Goodbye." We went to the reception room. He skipped over and took his mother's hand. "Hello there, Mother," he said. "I'm not coming back anymore." This today was for good-bye.

They left together—a little boy who had the opportunity to state himself through play and who had emerged a happy, capable child, and a mother who had grown in understanding and appreciation for her very gifted child.

Virginia Axline

Axline's classic, *Dibs*, provides an inspirational description of the ideal termination session. It was a planned termination that had been agreed upon by Dibs, his parents, and Dr. Axline after Dibs had made significant progress in treatment. By the close of his therapy, Dibs' initial symptoms had disappeared and he was functioning at an age-appropriate level. During the pretermination phase, Dibs showed signs that he had internalized the accepting and soothing functions of his therapist. He used several sessions to anticipate and mourn the ending of his therapy and was able to communicate and work through separation issues. His sense of self was stronger and he was clearly able to continue the process of development without further treatment. While Axline did not focus on transference or counter-transference issues, she was certainly empathically attuned and continually examined and monitored her personal reactions to Dibs. This served to keep her focus on his internal world and his therapeutic needs.

Axline's goal in describing this case was to provide a model for conducting child-centered play therapy. While her theory of the curative process is quite different from that of psychodynamic play therapists, this case clearly illustrates several of the issues and criteria referred to in the psychoanalytic literature on termination. These have been outlined by Parsons (1990) and include developmental considerations; strengthening the ego's functioning; the processes of mourning, internalization, and identification; resolving transference; and monitoring personal and countertransferential issues.

Parson's list can be used as a set of criteria to assess progress, the direction of treatment, and appropriate timing of the termination process. All of these issues are very much interrelated and will take on various forms and degrees of importance from case to case. Each of them requires careful consideration with regard to deciding whether the child is ready to end treatment and what issues might come up during the pretermination phase. These criteria will be considered separately in the interest of clarity.

DEVELOPMENTAL CONSIDERATIONS

There is in every child at every stage a new miracle of vigorous unfolding, which constitutes a new hope and a new responsibility for all.

Erik Erikson

Much of the literature dealing with the topic of termination in child psychotherapy has been provided by psychoanalysts and therapists who adhere to a developmental model. The issue of termination is seen as integrally related to the child's stage of development and to the assessment of whether treatment has helped to get the child to the point where progressive developmental forces can take over. However, it is clearly very difficult to determine when such a change has taken place, how it came about, and whether other latent fixations, conflicts, regressions, or problems remain. Thus deciding on the ideal time to terminate treatment with children is often difficult.

Van Dam and colleagues (1975) note that the dilemma of too little or too much treatment is of great importance when working with children. For some children, ending treatment can free them from regressive pulls and thereby allow the progress that has been made in treatment to integrate with age-appropriate developmental forces. For other children, ongoing treatment may be necessary in order for progressive developmental forces to take over. Because of the complex nature of these issues, van Dam and colleagues note that a child's readiness for termination must be evaluated from what they call a "multiple aspect view" (p. 445). They advocate the use of Anna Freud's (1962) "Developmental Profile" during the initial phase of treatment, for which it was developed, and again during the pretermination phase of treatment. Using the assessment procedure in this way provides the clinician with an internal picture of the child and an opportunity to compare both qualitative and quantitative changes that have taken place during the course of treatment. Chapter Three will describe the Developmental Profile in detail, with a focus on its usefulness to assess readiness for termination.

EGO FUNCTIONING

> The business of analysis is to secure the best possible psychological conditions for the functioning of the ego; when this has been done, analysis has accomplished its task.
>
> Sigmund Freud

Anna Freud has highlighted the fact that most children who are in need of psychological treatment are experiencing stress related to development, stress related to the environment, and/or regression or progression stemming from disharmony between developmental lines. In each of these cases, the ego is not working efficiently to mediate the internal, developmental, or external demands that are placed on it. Paulina Kernberg (1991) has set forth the following ten criteria for assessing ego strength and readiness for termination.

Statements about the Therapist

Progress in treatment is indicated when the child's statements reflect that she or he has had an experience of being listened to and helped and has internalized the therapist's functions in this regard. The latter might be indicated when the child begins to anticipate what the therapist will say or demonstrates, through behavior or speech, an identification with the therapist. A greater capacity for self-observation, self-understanding and reality testing indicates that the child has an increased ability to work through his or her own difficulties. An increased use of humor and statements about the therapist's personality or behavior may also reflect emergence from the transference neurosis.

Therapist's Interventions

Within the psychodynamic framework, confrontation and clarification are used early on to facilitate the child's communication. Interpretation is used to bring meaning to the child's communications as treatment progresses. Thus increased use of interpretation during the final stage of treatment indicates that the child has been able to communicate and that she or he has the capacity for understanding and insight.

Perception of Treatment

As termination approaches the child will introduce more material from everyday life and engage in less fantasy play. There will be more discussion about future plans, reminiscing about past events in therapy, emotional reactions such as sadness about leaving the therapist, and a wish to remain important to the therapist. Kernberg observes that "all of these criteria involving the perception of treatment reflect a more integrated self concept. The child's ability to relate to the analyst as a separate person and to view the treatment experience within a total life context suggests a growing strength in his/her observing ego" (p. 329).

Quality of Communications

Progress in treatment is often demonstrated when the child can convey feelings, needs, and thoughts through words instead of actions. This reflects secondary thought process that allows the child to delay gratification, to contemplate options, and to problem solve.

Play and Dreams

Play is often the primary mode of communication in the therapy room. The themes and conflicts that are communicated, the child's style, and the overall quality of the child's play will therefore evolve as progress takes place. By the close of treatment it is hoped that the child's play will convey a sense of freedom from conflict, anxiety, and other factors that may have precipitated treatment. Likewise, increased malleability and problem-solving ability, potential for sublimation, age-expected social skills, and an ability to derive pleasure from play should be evident.

Affects

One of the goals of treatment is for the child to develop a broader range of affects and to learn to modulate and verbalize them in an appropriate manner. The ability to express gratitude and concern is an important indication of readiness for termination. These affects represent a high level of object relations and an ability to modulate aggression.

Sublimatory Behavior

The capacity to channel drives in a more comfortable, spontaneous and socially acceptable way is indicated by the development and sharing of new ideas and interests. This is suggested through play via involvement with toys, games, and the like.

Insight

Insight is often demonstrated in less direct ways with children than with adults. Humor and the ability to laugh about habits, mannerisms, and mistakes suggest self-awareness and a healthy self-acceptance without the need for denial. Likewise, empathy toward others indicates an attempt to understand others through self-understanding. Regardless of the way in which insight is conveyed, the ability for self-monitoring fosters self-understanding and can prevent the child from repeating problematic behaviors.

Defenses

Flexibility and adaptiveness with regard to defenses suggest that the child has an internal sense of strength and resourcefulness. For instance, one of the major issues among children with behavior disorders is that they make rigid use of the defense of externalization. Growth is clearly indicated when such youngsters are strong enough to take responsibility for their behaviors and actions and/or when they are able to employ more adaptive, helpful defenses to deal with anxiety.

Appearance and Behavior

A decrease in symptoms, pathological character traits, and acting out and increased evidence of age-appropriate behaviors are expected by the close of treatment. Behaviors, mannerisms, posture, and style of dress each provide information regarding the child's identity, self-image, and level of self-esteem. With a decline in symptoms and acting-out behavior children tend to feel less helpless, more self-assured, and better equipped to procede with development.

WORKING THROUGH MOURNING REACTIONS, TRANSFERENCE, AND COUNTERTRANSFERENCE

In child analysis, the patient's experiences of being abandoned, neglected, or separated from the mother play an important part in the child's reactions in terminating. The need to work through these responses and defenses against the loss of object is an integral part of the work of termination in child analysis. It requires working on the problem of the resolution of transference ties as well as on the tie to the real object.

Anna Freud

Child therapists must fulfill two major roles simultaneously. They must serve as a *new object* to meet the child's need for a healthy new experience and at the same time must serve as a *transference object* so that the child can work through internal conflicts. For this reason, the termination phase of treatment often elicits a wide variety of emotional reactions among child patients. The complexity and layers of such reactions stem from previous experiences involving loss and separation as well as from the actual loss of the therapist. It is often difficult to distinguish transferential reactions from those that are related to losing the therapist. However, the whole matter of ending treatment and the therapist's reactions to saying goodbye, whether personal or induced by the child, can play a role in blurring the therapeutic picture. Accordingly, we need to consider each of these influences: childhood mourning and the processes of internalization and identification, transference reactions, and both personal and countertransferential reactions of the child therapist.

Childhood Mourning

> Did someone say that there would be an end,
> An end, Oh an end, to love and mourning?
> > May Sarton

Loewald (1962, 1988) proposed that the mourning process is the most important aspect of termination. For him, mourning involves letting go of the valued relationship and internalization of it. The question of how, and even whether children mourn following the loss of a loved one has been long debated (Deutsch 1937, Furman 1964, Nagera 1970, Wolfenstein 1966, 1969). Deutsch (1937) believed that a child's ego is not developed enough to tolerate the pain of mourning. Nonetheless, it has been consistently noted that children tend to regress following the loss of a significant person. Sekaer and Katz (1986) introduced the term *childhood mourning* to highlight that children work through losses differently than do adults. That is, for each stage of development there is an optimum degree to which mourning is possible. The child's cognitive development, to a great extent, dictates the degree to which the child can comprehend a loss experience.

According to Sekaer and Katz, children very often understand the external facts of the loss but they simultaneously maintain contradictory ideas and fantasies that distort the reality of the situation. Regardless of the child's conscious actions and verbalizations, active exploration of the child's emotions and thoughts regarding termination is of great importance. For instance, it is very common for children to feel abandoned when treatment is coming to an end. This is true even when they initiate termination or are actively involved in the decision to leave treatment. Broaching this subject with children and providing them with a period for working though emotions related to feeling abandoned can be of tremendous help. This may involve the use of direct statements aimed at clarifying the child's confused ideas and fantasies.

The psychological processes of internalization and identification have been held to play a major role in mourning. Horowitz and his colleagues (1980) believe that internalization involves taking on the role that the lost object performed in order to compensate for the absence. Wolfenstein (1969) comments that the mourning process serves an adaptive function by freeing libidinal energy that was bound to the lost object. She notes that mourning entails transferring the positive feelings attached to the lost person by establishing new interpersonal ties or through the process of identification. With regard to the latter, by identifying in a constructive manner the children themselves replace the lost person.

It is important to note that not all children are capable of internalization. Pedder (1982) argues that children who have good enough mothering develop a good enough internal object. Even when threatened by later losses the child with a good enough internal object is capable of healthy mourning and adaptive internalizations of the object that is being lost. In contrast, children who do not experience such mothering have difficulty mourning when later losses occur.

Children in treatment who have lacked adequate mothering are provided with an opportunity to acquire a good enough internal object via the therapeutic relationship. The child can work through separation-individuation issues that were left unresolved. Consolidation of these issues during the termination phase can help the child develop a stable inner representation of the therapist to carry with him or her for comfort long after treatment has ended.

Weiss (1991) proposes that the therapist fulfills the role of a transitional object for the child during treatment. However, in contrast to Winnicott, who believed that transitional objects are given up when they are no longer needed, and to others who believed that transitional objects are internalized, Weiss argues that when treatment ends the therapist's role as transitional object undergoes a transformation. This transformation takes place "so that it continues to be socially acceptable to both the individual and those around him" (p. 266). According to this theory, the analyst is not given up at the time of termination. Instead, she or he serves as a transitional object via memories. Weiss observes that

> most of us do not accept identification with the analyst as an ideal solution to the analytic ending, yet we find it acceptable that the patient takes on the analyst's analytic mode of thinking, presumably for the purpose of continuing a self-analysis. But can a cognitive self-analysis take place without identification, without the shadowy presence of the figure of the analyst? And is self-analysis in the service of insight and ego expansion, or is it an attempt to be soothed by memories of the analyst, its function akin to that of the transitional object of infancy? [pp. 266–267]

The defense mechanisms that children most commonly use when dealing with issues of loss include denial, idealization, identification, and displacement. In contrast to adults, children tend to mourn "at a distance" by displacing their feelings onto toys, fictional characters, or other objects (Sakaer and Katz

1986, Wolfenstein 1966). Fantasies about the therapist and concerns about what will happen following termination can appear in a disguised form. Likewise, feelings of anger, rage, abandonment, sadness, disappointment, and ambivalence can be expressed in a safe manner that ensures the child that the connection with the therapist is not threatened. This premise highlights the important role that play can have in working through issues of loss and mourning when ending treatment.

Transference Reactions

> There was a child went forth every day,
> And the first object he looked upon, that object he
>   became,
> And that object became part of him for the day or a
>   certain part of the day,
> Or for many years or stretching cycles of years.
>   Walt Whitman

The term transference, as it pertains to psychodynamic treatment with children, refers to the way in which the child's views of both past and present objects are expressed in his or her relationship with the therapist. Transference can be expressed in perceptions, thoughts, fantasies, feelings, attitudes, or behaviors. Anna Freud (in Sandler et al. 1980) noted that, with children, there are four different forms that transference can take: transference of habitual modes of relating, transference of current relationships, transference of past experiences, and transference neurosis.

Transference of habitual modes of relating, also called *character transference*, is seen when the child relates in a habitual fashion to a whole category of people. An example is the child who does not trust adults and therefore anticipates being disappointed or abandoned by the therapist. Such themes typically emerge in imaginative play. One of the major tasks in treating such children is to establish a therapeutic relationship so that the child will come to see the therapist in a different way, thereby challenging the cognitive set in which all adults are untrustworthy. The therapist can use play material such as dolls, puppets, and action figures to convey messages to the child indirectly. Consolidation of this understanding via working through past disappointments, work with parents, and separating in a sensitive, emotionally attuned manner when terminating treatment can bring about significant emotional healing.

Transference of current relationship is seen when the child's preoccupation with people in his or her present life spills over, is displaced, or is extended to the therapist. Such spillovers can be largely reality based and can therefore give the therapist a good deal of information about the child's experience and mode of adaptation to a current life situation. Anna Freud (in Sandler et al. 1980) provides the example of a boy whose father started a new job, requiring time to be away from the child. The child subsequently became negative toward the therapist, especially on Fridays, just before their weekend break. Thus the anger brought about in the child's life was aroused when a similar situation took place in treatment.

Transferential reactions related to current relationships can emerge when the child is forced to leave
treatment because of a family move. In such cases the
child is forced to deal with many separations and
losses simultaneously. Children typically feel abandoned even when they are the ones leaving. Thus
feelings of being left, abandoned, unimportant and/or
uncared for may emerge in transference reactions
related to current relationships, in addition to feelings
directly related to losing the therapeutic relationship.
It is important to sort out the sources of the child's
reactions.

Transferences of past relationships are derivatives
of repressed material that often emerge as a result of
treatment. Anna Freud observes that reactions are
typically a combination of present reality (including
the real relationship with the therapist) and expressions of re-emerged wishes, memories, or fantasies.
With regard to termination, regression is a very common phenomenon. The ending of treatment evokes
feelings related to the loss of the therapist as well as
feelings related to previous losses. A re-emergence of
old symptoms and problematic behaviors that had
previously dissipated is not uncommon during the
termination phase of treatment. These symptoms or
behaviors are often expressions of the child's perceptions of "needing" the therapist in order to do well. In
addition, they can be repetitions of the child's past in
the transference relationship. Children who experience early losses, be they psychic or physical, often
adapt defenses to cope with feelings. These children
are often not brought to treatment until problematic

behaviors or symptoms arise. During the termination phase, when symptoms and defenses are revived in the transference relationship, their analysis can lead to a working through of original feelings related to loss, helplessness, and the like.

Transference neurosis refers to an intensified transference in which a major internal conflict is externalized, so that it is perceived to occur between the individual and the therapist. A primary characteristic of transference neurosis is that the patient becomes preoccupied with the therapist and his or her symptoms related to the conflict simultaneously dissipate or even disappear. The issue of whether a transference neurosis can develop with children remains questionable. Certainly it is of the utmost importance that therapists always examine their role and how it may be affecting any form of transference that is present. When therapist factors are ruled out, careful tracking of changes in the child's transferential reactions can provide invaluable information regarding progress and issues to be addressed in preparation for terminating treatment.

Personal Reactions

> The task, at least with children, is to repair, not to remake.
>
> Stanley Spiegel

The therapeutic relationship that allows the clinician an opportunity to become involved with the emotional experiences, disappointments, and challenges of the child can bring about a personal connection, often making the issue of when to terminate treatment unclear and difficult. This is especially true when the child's caretakers and/or environmental supports are ineffectual or uninvolved. Anna Freud noted that it is not uncommon for child therapists to maintain a wish to immunize child patients against future difficulties prior to ending treatment. This, of course, is not possible and can account for prolonged treatment.

Coppolillo (1988) likens this tendency to the struggle that parents have in "letting go" of their children and cites a father who describes an incident with his 3-year-old daughter. The child had had a fantasy of petting wild animals but was extremely disappointed following a frightening encounter with a snake at the zoo. The girl's father wrote:

> I experienced enormous protectiveness and a wish that I could buffer her from every future disappointment and hurt when she offered her love and experienced aggression or callousness in return. As I held and comforted her on a convenient bench, I realized with some sadness that I could not buffer her from the future. All I could do was to offer the best of my being in the present for her use in the future, and hope that the strength she developed could see her through. [Coppolillo 1988, pp. 332–333]

Clearly, countertransference can play a major role in psychodynamic therapy with children. It is important not to underestimate the child's progress and contribute to the treatment's becoming interminable or overestimate the child's progress and terminate too quickly. When the therapist prolongs treatment or begins to feel that a child may be ready for termination, personal reactions should be ruled out. This is especially true if the decision is emotionally charged or unusual in some way. Questioning the extent to which the child and/or parent is eliciting this response from the therapist, the extent to which the response stems from the therapist's own history or current life situation, and the extent of loss the therapist is experiencing in relation to the child, will provide much-needed clarity.

It is not uncommon for therapists to experience a wide range of emotions during the termination phase of treatment. Successful terminations will certainly bring about a sense of achievement and satisfaction, while unsuccessful ones may elicit feelings of frustration, anger, disappointment, regret, or relief. Many terminations, successful or not, give rise to sadness and can evoke issues related to separation, loss, and grief. These emotions, whether related personally to the child or to something in the therapist's own history that is elicited by the child, are quite appropriate. They must, however, be addressed in a clear manner that does not interfere with the goals of treatment. Therapy must remain "therapy" until the very end. Clearly, it is important that the therapist not act out his or her emotions about ending the treatment in the therapeutic relationship. According to Coppolillo,

> the psychotherapy of the child continues throughout the termination phase. Time out for leave taking,

indulging that from which the child had previously abstained, "unbending," self-revelation of the therapist, and other departures from neutrality, inquiry, understanding, and interpretation by the therapist, when indulged without understanding the significance of the activity, may undo some of the benefits the child has won from the treatment process. Of course, the therapist has been a "real person" to the child, and of course there will be some pain in leaving him. But if, in order to make up for this loss, the therapist creates "palship time," or loving periods which can be looked back upon as the child strolls down memory lane, he may miss some important opportunities for insights that may be available due to the process of separating. This does not mean that the termination phase must be characterized by stiffness or rigidity, but only that it must be guided by the same disciplined scrunity that obtained in the earlier parts of treatment. [p. 325]

Countertransferential reactions of the therapist can be used to understand children who may not be expressing their feelings and thoughts about ending treatment. It is not uncommon for children to insist that they have no reactions to termination. In such situations, when atypical emotions such as anger, sadness, loss, or boredom are experienced by the therapist, these can be used to broach the subject of whether the child is feeling similarly. This can be done through verbal inquiry or via symbolic play or art techniques. In either case, the need to help the child confront and work through issues related to separation, abandonment, and neglect is an integral part of the termination phase.

3

USING A DEVELOPMENTAL PROFILE TO DETERMINE READINESS FOR ENDING TREATMENT

> When a child's functioning at the beginning of his
> analysis is compared by means of the Profile, the
> analyst becomes aware of the many qualitative and
> quantitative changes . . .
>   Herman van Dam, Christophe Heinicke,
>   and Morton Shane

Anna Freud's (1962) Developmental Profile is multidimensional and includes information about the referral, symptoms, family and developmental history, environmental influences, and the genetic, structural, and dynamic interactions of the child's personality. Equal attention is given to all of the child's areas of functioning. Hence use of the profile at the beginning of treatment and during the pretermination phase allows the therapist to assess the qualitative and quantitative aspects of development that have occurred during the course of treatment. As van Dam and colleagues (1975) note, "by virtue of this broader and comprehensive viewpoint, much of what otherwise would remain preconscious in the analyst, his so-called clinical intuition, enters into his judgment about termination. Finally, he may discover and become aware of some of his own blind spots!" (p. 445).

Following is a breakdown of each area considered in the Developmental Profile, with particular focus on using it as what van Dam and colleagues call a "multiple aspect" instrument to assess readiness for termination.

PRESENTING PROBLEMS

Anna Freud notes that presenting problems among children often include arrests in development, progressions or regressions, inhibitions, and symptoms. An understanding of presenting problems can shed light on developmental forces and other underlying dynamics or sources of difficulty. Thus periodic consideration of presenting problems throughout the course of treatment is important when working with children to assess whether symptoms have shifted. For instance, presenting problems are usually related to social, cognitive, affective, or bodily functions. Social problems may be manifested in immature, aggressive, antisocial, oppositional, isolating, or sexual behavior. Disturbances related to cognition may include prococity, learning and memory problems, or thought disorders. Affective difficulties might include hypochondriacal behavior, anxiety, or depression. Disturbances revealed in bodily functions might be manifested in problems with eating, sleeping, bowel or bladder control, speech, or motility.

One of the most common reasons for premature termination is that parents and often children themselves base readiness for termination on symptom reduction. This criterion is often inconsistent with true therapeutic progress. Presenting problems may vanish or symptom substitution can take place before real progress is made. In some cases, symptoms may remain despite therapeutic progress. It is important for child therapists to work with parents to provide education and insight about shifts that commonly occur during treatment. This can be done in a manner that respects confidentiality when information is provided in a general manner and the therapist is able to clearly define his/her role as an educator regarding child development. While this education may not prevent some parents from terminating treatment prematurely, having information about the nature of symptoms may make it easier for them to return to therapy at a later time.

DESCRIPTION OF THE CHILD

Observations of the child's play during the initial phase of treatment and again during pretermination yields information about progress and changes in general appearance and manner, attachment and separation behavior, interpersonal skills, affective and mood states, ability to put words to thoughts and feelings, problem solving, coping and use of defenses, fantasy life, reality testing, object relations, self-confidence and self-esteem, self-soothing mechanisms, and ability to experience joy via play behavior. This information, together with the parents' and child's reports regarding academic, social, and emotional functioning can help the clinician determine whether the child is progressing in accordance with his or her developmental stage. When considering termination, it is important for the therapist to question whether the child will be able to progress through subsequent developmental stages given an average expectable environment, and whether treatment would be recommended if the child were to be seen for the first time at this point in time (P. Kernberg 1991).

FAMILY BACKGROUND AND PERSONAL HISTORY

Consideration of the home environment before and after treatment is very important in assessing readiness for termination. Van Dam and colleagues (1975) emphasize the fact that conflicts and difficulties experienced by children often have their roots in the parental relationship and the child's perception of it. In making the decision to terminate treatment it is important to consider the extent to which the conflicts have been resolved and whether they will be further resolved or, alternatively, accentuated in a maladaptive direction given the ongoing parental environment.

Before beginning treatment with children it is important to understand the child's biological, psychological, and social history, starting with prenatal development and working to the present. Information about the child's temperament, developmental milestones, positive and negative experiences, defenses, and coping skills contributes to understanding the presenting problem and to treatment planning. A comprehensive assessment of the parents' background and their historical and current relationship to each other and to the child gives valuable information about the psychological climate of the home. It also sheds light on possible messages or themes that the child has internalized over time and that may have relevance to his or her object relations and psychological difficulties. Information regarding how the child's parents were parented; their philosophy of parenting; their co-parenting style, motivations, and resistances; and their understanding of and connection to the child can be used to develop a treatment plan for work with the parents, which is more often than not an essential component of successful treatment.

Perfection in the child or in the home situation is certainly not a criterion for successful termination. However, determining the extent to which the home environment will be able to foster the child's growth and provide for his or her vulnerabilities and needs is an extremely important criterion when deciding whether ongoing treatment is needed. Children from abusive or neglectful families in which the parents are noncompliant with treatment may require ongoing therapy even after intrapsychic improvement is noted. This is often the case with court-referred children who, because of a lack of support and guidance, are at risk for various difficulties. In such situations the therapist may choose to continue treatment until the child develops healthy and supportive relationships outside of the home environment.

ENVIRONMENTAL INFLUENCES

When conducting a psychodynamic assessment it is important to explore the history and influences of all the child's significant relationships with siblings, extended family members, peers, teachers, and others. Likewise, changes and important experiences in the child's life, and an understanding of how she or he reacted to them, are relevant to understanding the child's intrapsychic world.

Assessment of changes in the child's interpersonal skills, selection of friends, and quality of relatedness with both peers and adults will be helpful in determining readiness for ending treatment. Specifically, whether the child relates at an age-appropriate level and is capable of genuine give and take and consideration for others is very important, especially if the child is entering preadolescence. Development of these skills and the ability to engage in satisfying interpersonal relationships will often help the child to decathect the therapist and to deal with issues of loss at termination. Parenthetically, one of the most natural ways for children to terminate treatment is for them to become involved with so many healthy and productive activities and relationships that they simply do not have the time or the need for treatment: they are back on their age-appropriate developmental track. This is especially true with school-age children, with whom the challenge of achieving a sense of industry and competence in academics and peer relations is of paramount importance (Erikson 1963). Likewise, one of the major criteria for successful termination with children entering adolescence is the turn toward new partnerships (Van Dam et al. 1975).

LIBIDINAL DRIVE DEVELOPMENT

Noting the child's phase of development both before and after treatment is an important criterion for planning termination. The key question here becomes whether the child has proceeded to the age-appropriate stage (i.e., oral, anal, phallic, latency, preadolescent, or adolescent) and has achieved phase dominance. Shifts in the child's interests and preferences during play therapy sessions and outside of treatment are good indications of phase dominance. For instance, symbolic play is much more prevalent among children during the anal and phallic stages, whereas game play, play with rules, and a striking lack of imaginative play is characteristic of latency children. A gradual moving away from childish games to more adult games such as chess, and/or an increased independence and assertiveness, often signifies the onset of adolescence.

Libido distribution is another area of consideration. For instance, the child's self-esteem, independence, sense of well-being, ability to neutralize aggression, and quality of object relations are all important indicators. Games are a useful tool for assessing how the child plays, wins, and loses. Children who must win or won't win manifest self-esteem issues. Likewise, children who require a great deal of reassurance or those who tend to overestimate their abilities usually lack an internal sense of confidence and well-being. Con-

versely, children who can derive a sense of gratification from their achievements and object relationships
without becoming overly dependent on external sources
may no longer need the therapeutic relationship. The
child's level of narcissism in relation to the therapist
and to peers and adults outside of treatment should
therefore be considered. Relational issues such as
object constancy can be examined via observations of
the child when she or he is separating from loved ones.
The therapist needs to assess the child's ability to make
and keep friends and the frequency and intensity of
peer contacts. With the onset of preadolescence, a look
at how the child relates to peers of the opposite sex
becomes increasingly important as well. Van Dam and
colleagues (1975) note that by the end of treatment
peer relationshps should have a quality of genuine give
and take and the child should have an increased level
of consideration for the partner. This is especially
important because of the loss of the real relationship
with the therapist at termination.

AGGRESSIVE DRIVE DEVELOPMENT

When assessing aggressive drive development the therapist considers the quantity and quality of manifest
aggression, determining whether the child's level of
aggression is age appropriate, how it is manifested,
whether it is directed internally or toward others, and
how it affects the child's overall functioning. Evidence
of increased ability to neutralize aggression and to

channel it in age-appropriate behaviors is important when planning termination.

EGO DEVELOPMENT

One of the primary goals of psychodynamic psychotherapy is the consolidation of ego strength so that the child can rise to the challenge of development. An ongoing assessment of the child's ego functions provides the clinician with a barometer of the child's coping skills, deficits, and level of adaptation. This is an essential aspect of the developmental profile for determining and monitoring treatment goals. The ego assessment includes an examination of: (1) autonomous ego functions such as sensation, perception, speech, intelligence, control of motility, memory, reality testing, and secondary thought process; (2) synthetic ego functions such as the ability to integrate and organize experiences; (3) preferred defenses, when and how they are used, their age appropriateness, and their efficiency for dealing with anxiety; (4) whether the child employs a variety of defenses or a restricted or rigid repertoire; (5) the degree to which the child has a balanced availability of defenses and affects; (6) the balance between progressive and regressive drive and ego forces; and (7) the overall quality of ego integration and its level of flexibility and consistency.

With regard to these criteria, the more flexible, resourceful, and open the child becomes with regard to trying new coping skills, and the more appropriate his or her expression of affect, the less the need for

continued treatment. Factors such as frustration tolerance, sublimatory potential, attitude to anxiety, and
progressive as opposed to regressive developmental
forces are especially important in the developmental
profile (A. Freud 1962, 1965). In general, if during the
pretermination phase of treatment the child's frustration tolerance remains low there is a risk that more
anxiety will be generated than the child will be able to
handle effectively; thus regression, defensive anxiety,
and symptom formation will likely occur. Conversely,
children who show an adequate frustration tolerance
will be equipped to maintain or recover equilibrium
more successfully. Likewise, children with the ability
to accept and enjoy substitute means of gratification
will be less likely to need pathological solutions (e.g.,
tantrums, withdrawal, regression, acting out) in order
to cope.

When children learn, as a result of therapy, to
master external and internal danger situations actively
there is not only evidence of a better balanced ego
structure, but an indication that treatment has been
helpful. These youngsters will be able to deal more
effectively with the demands of the environment without further treatment because of their higher level of
proactive behavior for problem resolution. Conversely,
children who continue to manifest fearfulness and
defensiveness will most likely need continued treatment.

Anna Freud (1962) emphasizes that progressive
developmental forces and regressive tendencies are
present in all children and can be deduced from
observing the child's struggle between the wish to grow

up and the reluctance to do so. She notes that when progressive developmental forces outweigh regression, "the chances for normality and spontaneous recoveries are increased; symptom formation is more transitory since strong forward moves to the next developmental level alter the inner balance of forces" (p. 157). Conversely, when regression outweighs progressive development, resistance and problematic solutions to difficulties impede therapeutic progress and indicate the need for additional treatment.

The child's attitude toward school, work, achievements, and the future, as well as his or her ability for self observation, are also important indicators of therapeutic progress. The goal of helping the child to resume the task of development clearly has a great deal to do with achievement and a positive and empowered feeling about the future.

SUPEREGO DEVELOPMENT

The degree to which the child's defenses and behaviors are dependent on others (the object world) or independent of them will give the clinician some sense of the child's superego development. Some considerations relevant to the termination phase include the extent to which the child internalizes or externalizes (i.e., the degree to which she or he experiences guilt as opposed to fear of the external world) and the child's internalization of a moral code. By the close of treatment it is important for children to have worked through unrealistic inner representations that adversely influenced superego development and for them to have developed a more realistic and practical understanding of the expectations of the real world.

GENETIC ASSESSMENTS (REGRESSION AND FIXATION POINTS)

Observations and history regarding the child's behaviors, fantasy activity, and symptomatology provide the clinician with information about regression and/or fixation points. Anna Freud (1962) notes that certain forms of manifest behavior that may be characteristic for a given child will provide an understanding of underlying id processes. She provides the examples of an obsessional child who is excessively clean and orderly and who has difficulties sharing, and whose fixation is therefore at the anal-sadistic phase; the excessively shy child who defends against exhibitionism; and the child with separation issues who is struggling with underlying ambivalence toward the caretaker. The extent to which these trouble spots are worked through and the extent to which there have been changes in the child's defenses for coping with them are yet other criteria for termination. Working with play materials can be particularly helpful for assessing the child's conscious and unconscious fantasies, which can be very telling regarding his or her developmental history.

Van Dam and colleagues (1975) point out that conducting genetic assessments of readiness for termination requires that the clinician recall the pattern of working through that occurred during the treatment. Focus is on the dominant conflicts, the sequence in which conflicts appeared, and the way in which these showed up in the transference. Working with this model allows the clinician to detect symptom substitution and prevents premature termination of treatment.

DYNAMIC AND STRUCTURAL ASSESSMENTS (CONFLICTS)

Establishing a good dynamic and structural understanding of conflicts early on is a useful methodology for determining whether treatment has been effective. Anna Freud (1965) proposed that structural conflicts usually take on one of three forms in children. Conflicts between the id or ego and demands of the external world arouse fear of the object world; conflicts between ego or superego and id impulses give rise to guilt; and conflicts stemming from insufficient fusion of competing drives manifest as ambivalence related to activity versus passivity, masculinity versus femininity, or the like.

With regard to planning termination, the extent of conflict present in the child and the extent to which it adversely affects his or her functioning becomes a key issue. As conflicts are resolved the child's anxiety tends to diminish and there tends to be a higher level of ego autonomy and efficiency in coping and problem solving. Qualitative observations of the child commonly reveal a greater degree of internal freedom, sponaneity, and self-confidence. Conflicts may still be present, but these do not impede the child's functioning, interpersonal relationsips, or sense of self.

PERSONALITY CHARACTERISTICS

While parent and teacher reports regarding improvements in the child's behavior are often important considerations, the timing of termination is best determined by the child and the therapist who are attuned to the child's subjective states and internal world. Coppolillo (1988) describes the changes that occur in the therapeutic process as the child becomes free from conflict and better able to relate to others. The child becomes more interesting and likeable to the therapist. She or he is no longer so preoccupied with anxiety or the avoidance of it that he ignores the rest of the world. As such, the child's interests and interpersonal connectedness expand. In response, the therapist may feel less need to support the child because of the child's increased security. The therapist can discuss a problem with the child and no longer needs to demonstrate that it exists. This indicates that defenses are more fluid. Due to the resolution of ambivalences, the child's affection springs more spontaneously from attachment rather than loneliness or fear. Sessions with the child are frequently experienced by the therapist as pleasant and the child is less resistant and more interpersonally connected.

Each child is unique and will require special attention regarding his/her readiness for termination. However, Coppolillo has identified several observable traits that are common indicators of successful treatment. These include:

1. The child begins to demonstrate a clear and firm sense of self. S/he is able to discern her/his beliefs and wishes from the attitudes and wishes of others.
2. The child can contemplate a variety of options for responding or adapting to the demands of the environment.
3. Freedom from symptoms is maintained as a result of the working through process.
4. Age-appropriateness is noted in the child's play behavior, interests, and the way s/he relates to peers. The child can use regression but is no longer dominated by it.
5. The child is able to observe her/his own behavior.
6. The child perceives the environment with more positive expectations and decreased anxiety.
7. The child comes to feel more positive about the world and enjoys age-appropriate activities and interpersonal relationships.

After treatment children often become less defensive and more engaging. There is less need for externalization and avoidance because of an increased level of self-acceptance. With this often comes a better sense of humor and higher level of self-esteem. Coppolillo notes that in general, children become more likeable to the therapist and to the interpersonal world because they are easier to be with.

PART TWO

PLANNED ENDINGS FOLLOWING SUCCESSFUL TREATMENT

Values from any life experience retain their positive meaning only as the individual is free to use them in the ever-recurring newness of living.

Frederick Allen

4

ENDING TREATMENT WITH CHILDREN WITH CHILDREN BETWEEN 3 AND 5

In the act of play, a child may discover a connective bridge between his isolation and the therapist's empathic understanding.

Howard Robinson

Children between the ages of 3 and 5 are frequently referred to as prelatency children or preschoolers. These terms will be used interchangeably in this section.

Under normal circumstances the child of 3 is approaching or already in the oedipal stage of development, is well on the way to object constancy, and is beginning to demonstrate superego development. Erikson (1963) observed that during this stage the child is confronted with the challenge of initiative (instigated by new locomotor and mental powers) versus guilt (for having "big ideas").

Prelatency children can develop an attachment to the therapist despite their strong ties to caretakers. However, they may have difficulties accepting the therapist's point of view because of the age-appropriate cognitive limitations that Piaget (1951) characterized as "egocentricity." Likewise, the prelatency child may have difficulty understanding the therapist's verbalizations. The therapist must therefore be careful to speak to the child in a manner that is within the child's range of ability and experience (Glenn 1978). For the preschool child the most meaningful level of communication is the language of play.

Perhaps the most striking feature of children between 3 and 5 is the prevalence and richness of their symbolic play. Psychoanalysts believe that symbolic play incorporates creative displacements, condensations, and representations of primary process thought and thus reveals the child's fantasy life (Glenn 1978) as well as current life events (Solnit 1987). Through such symbolic expressions the preschool child vicariously experiences and expresses emotions, concerns, and conflicts that she or he cannot acknowledge directly. The challenge for therapists working with prelatency children is to provide an arena for such expression, to make sense of the child's symbolic communications, and to help the child confront and work through issues by means of the metaphor of play.

TAILORING PLAY AND ART THERAPY
TECHNIQUES AND MATERIALS

The most essential aspect of treatment with the preschooler is the development of a play language with which to communicate. This occurs through joining the child's symbolic play and following his or her directions as to how to act out a role, who to be, where to move or hide, how loudly to speak, what to draw, and so forth. Creating such a play dialogue, wherein the therapist becomes the "actor" of the child's fantasies, allows for an elaboration of the child's symbolic play. The therapist stays within the play metaphor and first makes comments about conscious, surface issues. The therapist may also ask questions to help the child elaborate and paint a picture of themes. Later, as treatment progresses, interpretation of issues pertaining to unconscious fantasies, thoughts, and feelings takes place. In general, defenses are pointed out before content or drive (Glenn 1978).

As noted earlier, Paulina Kernberg (1991) lists increased use of interpretation by the therapist as an important indicator of therapeutic progress. This suggests that the child is able to communicate and that she or he has the capacity for understanding and insight. One exception to this might occur when the child is defending against feelings or thoughts pertaining to the termination itself or to concerns about previous losses or separations that are prompted by termination.

It is important to have a wide variety of toys with symbolic expressive value in the playroom or office throughout treatment. During termination, toys for working through separation and individuation issues are particularly important. In the interest of clarity I have divided these into six general and overlapping categories.

Toys for expression of mobility include automobiles, trucks, airplanes, helicopters, boats, hot-air balloons, and the like. These are essential for working through issues related to arriving and leaving, separation and reunion, loss, rejection, abandonment, and withdrawal.

Toys for expression of freedom include butterflies, birds (with multiple nests), wild animals and wild animal families, keys, handcuffs, and good guy/bad guy action figures. These can be helpful for resolving issues related to feeling "bad," rejected, or abandoned; letting go; withdrawing; fear and anxiety about being alone; and internalizing therapeutic gains.

Toys for expression of nurturance such as dolls, baby bottles, doctor kits, and stuffed animals are useful for representing themes related to self-soothing and internalization of the comforting elements of treatment. Mahler and colleagues (1975) have noted that the role playing that is common during the final stage of separation-individuation serves to strengthen the ego, allowing a greater tolerance for separation and an identification with adults.

Toys for connecting and relating include interaction- and communication-oriented toys such as costumes, hats, cooperative games, telephones, and walkie-talkies. These toys allow for role playing and help the child to use the therapist as the rapprochement child uses the caretaker, for refueling to further the separation process. Nerf-ball catch, telephones, and walkie-talkies are particularly useful for themes related to connecting and letting go. It is important to have two telephones so that the therapist can "connect" and convey that the child is "heard." Binoculars are also useful for issues pertaining to closeness, safety, and feelings about the therapist. Finally, cameras are extremely important for noting when a child wants to hold on to a moment or memory.

Toys for expression of growth and self-esteem such as birds, butterflies, or silk flowers are useful for addressing issues related to "blossoming" and new-found autonomy, independence, and self-esteem. Gems, jewelry and colored coins can also be used to address issues of self-worth, dignity, and individuality. Finally, make-believe crowns are useful for empowerment work (Johnson 1996).

Other important toys include a doll house, domestic animals and animal families, monsters to address fears, a magic wand, a bop bag to address anger, sunglasses and masks to address withdrawal or hiding themes, play money to address issues related to "being paid for," and art supplies such as clay, beeswax, small and large sheets of drawing paper, markers, crayons, and colored pencils. The art materials are useful as supplements to each of the categories described above.

CASE ILLUSTRATION

Presenting Problem and Background

Michelle was 4 years, 11 months old when she was brought for treatment by her mother. She was an only child whose family had relocated to the area two months earlier. Michelle had become increasingly defiant and difficult since the move. She reportedly "played cat and mouse games" with her mother, would dart away in public places and hide, or hide at home when mom instructed her to do something. When disciplined for this behavior, Michelle would scream, pull her hair, and sometimes run away. While she reportedly enjoyed being with other children, her nursery school teacher reported that Michelle was "bossy" and would get mad at her peers quite easily.

Michelle's birth was unplanned by her parents, who had been dating for just over a year when she was conceived. They were reportedly happy, albeit shocked and unprepared for the pregnancy. Nonetheless, they married and settled into the role of parents without much difficulty.

Four months after Michelle's birth, Mr. D's company transferred him out of state. Mrs. D., having left her job and graduate school program to be a full-time mother, moved with him. However, she found it hard to be away from her family and friends and began to cling to Michelle. At this time she became "overinvolved and overprotective" and would not "let Michelle out of sight." Michelle resisted her mother's protectiveness and by 18 months would dart away from her in public places. This caused Mrs. D. extreme anxiety about the possibility that Michelle would be kidnapped or lost and served to exacerbate maternal worry and overprotectiveness.

When Michelle was 2 ½ years old her father was transferred to Europe for a one-year assignment with his firm. Mrs. D. decided not to accompany her husband and remained in their home with Michelle. Mr. D. visited the family one to two times a month for periods of two to five days. During this time Michelle became "overly attached" to her mom and "distant" from her dad. During his visits, she would compete with her dad for mom's attention and would throw tantrums when dad attempted to join or take over rituals such as bath time or story time. The tantrums entailed pulling her hair, screaming, stamping her feet, and at times running out to the street. The latter caused panic in Mrs. D., who feared that Michelle would be hit by a car.

Shortly after Mr. D. completed his work in Europe he was promoted to a permanent position on the east coast. Mrs. D. was upset that she would have to relocate and start over again. Reportedly, Michelle was also unhappy about the move.

Early and Middle Phases of Treatment

Michelle presented as a strikingly appealing child who was large in stature and slightly overweight for her age. She demonstrated very advanced verbal, gross, and fine motor skills and carried herself in a confident, precocious manner. She separated easily from her mother during the first session and throughout most of her treatment.

Michelle was very independent during our early sessions and always chose to do things alone such as looking through the toys, opening and closing containers, putting toys away, and the like. There was an air of "don't get in my way" about her. Nonetheless, she enjoyed toys that required interaction with the therapist such as having tea parties, playing Candyland, and taking turns changing dolls. Before long she began to treat the therapist just as she reportedly treated her agemates. She was bossy and quick to change her mind. For instance, she would instruct the therapist to put an outfit on a doll and would abruptly pull the doll away because she changed her mind about the outfit or she simply wanted to do it herself.

Michelle engaged in minimal symbolic play for several weeks. However, by the middle of the second month of treatment she would begin most sessions by playing with the doll house. Two major themes emerged during the remainder of her treatment and were worked through via the metaphor of symbolic play.

The first theme, which emerged in the fifth session and was repeated intermittently throughout the second, third and fourth months of treatment, involved the father doll drowning. Michelle's dramatization of this event was emotionally charged. The scenario involved a family going on a rafting trip, the father falling out of the raft and screaming for help, and the child (either boy or girl) attempting to help but failing. The father then drowns. Each dramatization of this play theme was followed by rapid movement to a different scene such as dinner time with the whole family, including the father, or to a different toy.

Michelle's play expressed her struggle with how to integrate her father into her world and back into the family. This play allowed her, in a safe and disguised manner, to express her wish to be rid of him as well as her anxiety about losing him. She was working through abandonment issues related to his unpredictable absences earlier in her life. In play, Michelle was in charge of her father's presence, absence and survival. Another level of this theme was the issue of "an accident." Michelle's mother was very concerned about Michelle's safety and frequently warned her to be careful. This play theme allowed Michelle to work through anxiety which was ever-present in her interactions with mom.

The second theme involved Michelle's repeated tendency to put either the little girl or the little boy doll in the closet with the door shut closed. Michelle would continue to play with the other dolls but would keep the child in the closet throughout her dramatization. Over time, the child in the closet emerged as a representation both of Michelle's sense of being out of control and needing to contain her impulses and of her sense that she was confined and stifled by her mother's overprotectiveness.

Michelle's defense of controlling and bossing helped her to deal with feelings of vulnerability resulting from anxiety and anger about being confined by her mother. She acted out these feelings by taking on the role of the controlling, aggressive, and at times sadistic member of the mother–daughter dyad (the sadistic element being represented, for example, by her hiding or running into the street to panic her mother). This role left Michelle with a sense of being out of control. Thus, by keeping a doll in the closet, she was able to contain and gain control of her angry impulses and gradually to work through her deeper issue of being confined. Through repetitive play she became master of a situation that she had previously experienced in a passive manner. The battle of "control or be controlled" was no longer necessary at home, as mom also learned more effective ways to cope.

Work with Michelle's Parents

Anna Freud (1965) wrote, "It is not the patient's ego but the parents' reason and insight on which beginning, continuance, and completion of treatment must rely" (p. 48). This section is included to highlight the important role that Michelle's parents played throughout her treatment, especially during the termination phase.

Mr. and Mrs. D. were seen bimonthly for parent counseling that was used to address the family dynamics, which were in a state of flux because of Mr. D's reunion with the family. Counseling focused on redefining his role as a full-time parent and a support to Mrs. D, on developing effective co-parenting skills, and on Michelle's feelings about his presence and previous absence. Control issues played out between Michelle and her mom were also discussed in great detail. Mrs. D. realized that these battles resonated with issues from her relationship with her own mother, who was also overprotective. She sought individual therapy to address them during the sixth month of Michelle's treatment.

By the ninth month of treatment, Mr. D. had established himself as a stable, consistent, and very loving parent to Michelle. Likewise, Mrs. D. made significant progress with regard to avoiding power struggles. Michelle's behaviors had also improved dramatically. She was less bossy and aggressive and displayed significantly fewer defiant behaviors and tantrums. When she did get upset and willful, she was able to calm down much more quickly. These changes coincided with developmental changes signifying that Michelle was approaching latency.

Over a period of several weeks, Michelle had been expressing a desire to stop treatment before she started first grade. The developmental profile, which was used before and after treatment, showed significant progress in Michelle's ego functioning. Improvements were noted in her ability to tolerate frustration, self-soothe, neutralize aggression, entertain options and compromises, and sublimate in difficult situations. Although Michelle was back on an age-appropriate developmental track, there was concern regarding her handling of termination because of her history of repeated separations from dad. I expressed this concern to Mr. and Mrs. D. and they fully supported a gradual period of termination and working through.

Termination Phase

As I have noted, Coppolillo (1988) believes that one indication that treatment may no longer be needed is that the child becomes more likeable to the therapist. This was certainly the case with Michelle. She was more interpersonally connected, significantly less bossy and domineering, and better able to engage in cooperative play. Overall, Michelle presented as less egocentric and defensive, and more spontaneous and trusting. She no longer needed to be in charge of everything as she knew that the therapist would not try to control her.

The decision to terminate Michelle's treatment was made during our thirty-eighth session. After saying that we would end treatment, I emphasized that we would need some time to say goodbye. Michelle just nodded. She proceeded to play with the doll house, then with the school, and later with the hospital. There were no notable themes to the play and Michelle appeared somewhat removed. She was setting up scenarios with the play materials but did not seem truly involved with the play. Likewise, she quickly lost interest in the scenarios and shifted from one play theme to another. I sat next to Michelle throughout the session but she did not include me in her play. She seemed somewhat overwhelmed and appeared to be grappling with how to use her sessions and how to relate to me. I commented about this and stressed the fact that she could use the four remaining sessions however she would like.

Michelle arrived for the next session in good spirits. She promptly took out the Jenga game, and as soon as we finished playing it she bounced up, put it away, and took out a second game for us to play. When we finished playing that game, Michelle again bounced up and chose a third game. This pattern continued throughout the session. By the middle of this meeting it became apparent that Michelle had given some thought as to how she would use this session. She was somehow reviewing each of the games we had played throughout our work together. I joined her in this reminiscence by attempting to connect memories to the games she chose. For instance, when we played Candyland I commented that it was the first game we had played together. Likewise, when we played The Sleeping Grump, I noted that we had played it on her birthday. Michelle and I played a total of seven different games during this session. There was a strong sense of connectedness and of letting go—a feeling that Michelle was attempting to look back at the road we had traveled together.

Michelle played with rubber stamps and an ink pad during the following session. She tried out each stamp to see how it would look on the drawing paper. She talked briefly about her upcoming visit to her grandmother's house, but overall she was significantly less interactive during this session. It appeared that she was taking a break from the work of mourning and letting go and was using the session to explore new skills. Her level of curiosity, initiative, and industry with the rubber stamps was quite striking.

Michelle's parents reported that she had become increasingly clingy with her mother over the following week. When I greeted her for our next session, I found Michelle standing next to her mom, leaning her head across mom's shoulder. She entered the play room willingly, but her movements were slow and deliberate, as though she were lacking energy. Michelle took out the two baby dolls and began to focus on feeding them and then changing their outfits. She then put on an apron and proceeded to cook stew. The theme of taking care of the babies while being busy cooking emerged. Michelle talked about what she was doing but did not include me in this play. She seemed to be testing out her resources for nurturing, soothing, and coping.

It appeared that a sense of mastery was achieved through this play. Michelle took off her apron after putting the babies down for a nap and finishing dinner. She then put on several "crystal" necklaces and a hat to prepare herself for dinner. Her use of the jewels revealed a sense of self-worth and dignity. I pointed out that she had worked hard and could now feel good about all she did. This comment was made about the play scene but was intended as a general metaphorical statement about Michelle's work in therapy. She left the session in a much more animated fashion and cheerfully greeted her mother in the waiting room.

Michelle brought her own baby doll to her last session and kept it by her side while she drew a picture of a house. Although she had brought this doll to previous sessions, its presence during the termination phase suggested that it was being used as a transitional object. As I watched Michelle handle the doll, it occurred to me that she would be leaving therapy but she would not be leaving alone.

While drawing, Michelle spontaneously mentioned that the picture was of her grandmother's house, and she discussed her upcoming visit to her grandmother, the fact that the family would take an airplane to get there, and so on. At one point she asked for my assistance in drawing a squirrel. It seemed that Michelle wanted me to contribute to her drawing as she instructed me to put the squirrel on the tree in the picture. When it was time to say goodbye, Michelle put the drawing supplies away and asked whether she could take the picture home with her. I said, "Of course" and stressed that it would be a nice souvenir of our last session together. Michelle smiled and left the session as she did all sessions. She simply said, "Bye, Donna" and proceeded to greet her mother in the waiting room with her usual animated skip.

Michelle had used the termination period of her treatment to acknowledge the reality of an ending, to reminisce about our work together, to test out her internal resources, to work through her sense of mourning related to letting go, and to reflect on future events. She had internalized the soothing elements of treatment and had progressed to latency. The latter was indicated in her behavior and increased verbal ability. It is interesting to note that Michelle's drawing was characteristic of what we find in a latency-age child. There was significantly less fantasy and its neatness and structure suggested age-appropriate repression and focus on reality. Her general demeanor and her emphasis on the upcoming family vacation and visit to grandma's revealed that she now saw mom, dad, and herself as a unit. There was a sense of hopefulness and adventure about the future.

5

ENDING TREATMENT
WITH CHILDREN
BETWEEN 6 AND 10

[T]he urge to do theatre is a very natural thing. It stems from the urge to play that exists in all of us. As we grow we have to funnel this urge into other forms.

Bar-Ya'cov

Children between the ages of 6 and 10 are frequently referred to as latency or school-age children. These terms will be used interchangeably throughout this section.

According to psychoanalytic theory, latency follows the passage of the oedipal phase and the establishment of the superego. The latency stage, under nomal circumstances, is marked by the repression, desexualization, inhibition, and sublimation of libidinal impulses (Schechter and Combrinck-Graham 1980). With the resolution of oedipal issues, the ego is freed so the child can focus on the world outside of the family, namely on the world of school and peer relations (Erikson 1963).

Erikson (1963) emphasized the challenge of establishing a sense of industry as the paramount feature of this phase of development. He noted that successful completion of this stage requires that the child focus on learning and functioning in the outside world. If the child is still preoccupied with issues related to the family, she or he is not free to learn the skills of society such as reading, writing, arithmetic, and interpersonal functioning. The unfortunate result is a sense of incompetence and inferiority.

Repression and other defenses including reaction formation, sublimation, fantasy, and obsessive-compulsive features are characteristic of this stage and allow the child to stay focused on the developmental task of achieving a sense of competence and mastery. Erna Furman (1980) notes that externalization is also commonly used by latency-age children to ward off inner conflict. She writes:

> . . . the child relegates the superego function to a potential authority whom he then defies but whom he also "invites" to control or punish the displayed misdeeds. This externalization, like projection, thus has the feature of tying the patient to the person onto whom he externalizes and from whom he expects criticism. However, the externalization not only changes an inner battle into an outer one; it also supplants a very harsh inner threat with a usually milder punishment from the outside. Further, the "crime" is often displaced; e.g., naughty behavior may be shown instead of a guilt-provoking masturbatory activity. [p. 271]

Externalization is evident in children who are afraid of monsters, the dark, evil spirits, and the like (Novick and Kelly 1970).

At the age of 6 or 7 the child enters the stage of concrete operations, which is marked by the use of logic that is bound to objects and situations. The child becomes less egocentric, more verbal, and increasingly capable of seeing things from the point of view of others (Piaget 1951, Schechter and Combrinck-Graham 1980). Nonetheless, the latency child's concreteness and level of repression makes treating these youngsters a challenging task. The therapist needs to be attuned to the child's constantly changing needs and modes of communication. In describing the latency period, Melanie Klein (1932) wrote:

> Unlike the small child, whose lively imagination and acute anxiety enable us to gain an easier insight into its unconscious and make contact there, they [latency children] have a very limited imaginative life, in accordance with the strong tendency to repression which is characteristic of their age; while, in comparison with the grown-up person, their ego is still undeveloped, and they neither understand that they are ill nor want to be cured, so that they have no incentive to start analysis and no encouragement to go on with it. [p. 94]

TAILORING PLAY AND ART THERAPY TECHNIQUES AND MATERIALS

Glenn (1978) notes that the latency child's narcissism decreases and his object orientation increases throughout this stage of development. There is clearly a movement away from nonverbal, imaginative play to more verbal play during early latency and finally to direct verbal communication with the therapist by late latency and preadolescence (Maenchen 1970). While symbolic play continues through much of the latency period, it tends to decrease as time goes by. Simultaneously, there is a gradual increase in verbalization and an interest in project-oriented toys and games with rules. When these games are spontaneous and invented, an underlying symbolic theme can commonly be understood and used by the therapist. Likewise, when games with rules are played, the child's aim and the ways in which the game allows for winning or losing can be used to understand underlying dynamics, fantasies, and themes (Solnit 1987).

During the termination phase of treatment it is not uncommon for latency children to complain of being bored and of having nothing to talk about, and to protest that there is no need to continue treatment. They commonly deal with their feelings by using structured games defensively, that is, to ward off, hide, or disguise feelings and fantasies. Such a use of games is not to be confused with genuine play. To the contrary, this defensive use of play is much more characteristic of resistance and/or emotional withdrawal from treatment. It needs to be confronted and interpreted so that the restricted, resistant, or overwhelmed child can move to age-appropriate play, which will promote the working through of separation issues (Solnit 1987).

Despite the developmental differences of latency and prelatency children, it is important to keep in mind that themes of separation and individuation will re-emerge during the termination phase of treatment with all age groups. Therefore, toys that promote themes of mobility, freedom, relating and connecting, nurturance, growth, and self-esteem, which were described in the previous chapter, can be useful for latency children during termination. However, it is important to have toys appropriate to the intellectual and developmental level of latency children available as well. For instance, latency-stage children are typically very interested in projects such as drawing a picture, building a castle, making a story book, constructing a tunnel, developing a floor plan, and the like. They can become absorbed in such activity with great intensity. The therapist can use the metaphor of the "project" to address what is going on with the child. A wide variety of art and drawing supplies as well as constructive toys such as Legos, Fiddle Sticks, and various sizes and shapes of blocks are essential for the latency child's "project play."

With disorganized or timid children, or those who are seen on a short-term basis, the therapist may choose to structure the termination phase by introducing a project to be worked on in preparation for the final session. Examples would include drawing a coat of arms with four to six sections for pictures about themes discussed in treatment, building a box in which to keep special memories or thoughts, or making a collage depicting things learned in therapy. These and other techniques are described in the Appendix.

Board and card games can be used very productively with latency children as they provide an anchor for physical activity, limit the pull to regressive behavior, and simultaneously remove the child's self-consciousness, thereby permitting him or her to communicate more comfortably. In this sense they serve the same function as toys that allow for relating and connecting.

Finally, the more verbal techniques of role playing, making up stories and plays, and using therapeutic board games can address issues related to separation, abandonment, rejection, anxiety, individuation, and freedom.

CASE ILLUSTRATION

Presenting Problem and Background

Terri, a 9-year-old girl with anxiety and adjustment difficulties, was previously described by this author (Cangelosi 1995). The child was brought for treatment by her mother and stepfather because of anxiety related to separating from her mother, nightmares, insomnia, and a pattern of becoming tearful and agitated at bedtime. These symptoms appeared one month prior to the initial parent consultation. They were first noted during a weekend visit with her natural father. This was the first time that Terri spent the night at his house since his girlfriend Kathy had moved in with him. Terri became so upset on that particular night that Kathy decided to sleep with Terri to comfort her. When Terri returned home after the weekend her symptoms continued and began to generalize to the point that she sometimes followed her mother around the house. Terri's mother, Mrs. G., was so upset by the child's panic and fear that she set up a cot in Terri's bedroom.

At the time of the initial consultation, Mrs. G. had not slept in her own bedroom for over three weeks. Interestingly, it was just six weeks before the symptoms began that Terri was informed that her mother and stepfather were going to have a baby. Terri, who had been an only child for nine years, reportedly took the news very well and verbally welcomed the idea of being a big sister. Nonetheless, Mrs. G. noted that Terri had become increasingly withdrawn since she was told about the baby.

The developmental history revealed that Terri had not demonstrated any difficulties with separations earlier in her life. Her parents divorced when she was 3 years old and she had lived alone with her mom for over five years. Mrs. G. dated Mr. G. for over four of these five years and he developed a very close relationship with Terri during that time. Nonetheless, after the marriage (eight months before treatment began) Terri became somewhat withdrawn and complained of not liking it when her stepfather told her what to do. At the same time, she was described as being very affectionate toward him. Terri's relationship with her biological father was described as "consistently inconsistent." There was no set visitation pattern and he frequently did not call Terri for weeks at a time. In spite of this, Mrs. G. noted that she made sure to maintain a relationship with her ex-husband so that she would always be able to talk with him about Terri.

Early and Middle Phases of Treatment

Terri arrived for her first session accompanied by her mother. When I greeted them in the waiting room, Mrs. G. was extremely anxious; she confided that Terri did not want to come to the session but that they had worked out "a deal." Terri then came into the therapy room without hesitation. She seemed very tense and uncomfortable and informed me that she had nothing to talk about and had come only because she wanted to go to the mall afterward. I responded to Terri by saying that it must be hard when parents make so many decisions. Terri nodded and looked down. I sensed that she had made up her mind not to talk about this matter further, and so I proceeded to show her the cabinet of toys and art supplies. I told her that even though she didn't choose to come to see me, she could choose what to do. Terri sheepishly took out paper and a pencil and began to draw a house.

She became absorbed with the drawing and embellished it with meticulous detail. She added fancy doorknobs, curtains, window panes, a cobblestone walkway, and then a flower-trimmed garage and mailbox. A smiling girl, with the same degree of detail, was drawn with a letter in her hand that she was mailing. The girl was trimmed with lace and topped off with a flowered hat. Even her shoes and the letter had bows on them. Scenery was added behind the house. Snow-capped mountains, trees, birds, and a sun filled the sky. A raccoon with disproportionately large eyes (and eyelashes) was drawn peeking out of one of the trees. Throughout the time that Terri drew this picture I occasionally commented or asked questions. For instance, when the raccoon was drawn, I noted that raccoons stay up at night. I also inquired about the letter the girl was mailing but Terri simply responded that it was "just a letter."

Terri became increasingly relaxed and animated as the session and the drawing progressed. The session closed on a much more positive note than the one on which it had begun. Afterward, I noted to myself that Terri was dressed in much the same way as the girl in her picture, that is, with meticulous detail, and this was, in fact, a pattern in the weeks that followed. Terri arrived each week in a different outfit with matching socks, shoes, purses, belts, and hair ornaments. While some of this concern with appearance could be seen as age appropriate, it was Terri's obsessive defense and extremely high standards that stood out as ongoing themes throughout her treatment. The high standards seemed to reflect the superego demands characteristic of the latency period. On the basis of Terri's developmental history and overall presentation, I suspected that her fears and anxieties were at least in part a result of harsh, externalized superego demands.

Terri used many sessions to draw or to make craft projects. She consistently demonstrated a need to include obsessive detail in these projects and frequently concealed them from me to make sure that they turned out the way she wanted. When they did not, Terri became frustrated and complained vehemently that it was "stupid coming to therapy." These instances were used to address Terri's use of externalization. I frequently pointed out that Terri thought everyone expected as much from her as she did. Throughout the first few months, the focus was on helping her to discriminate between what she expected of herself and what others expected of her.

By the second month of treatment Terri demonstrated more and more anger toward me. She consistently started each session by complaining about having to come to therapy and then proceeded to discuss concerns while becoming involved in art projects. Therapy provided a safe arena for her to express anger. During one session she used rubber stamps to make a picture of a family walking together. A baby was in the picture, separated from the rest of the family and suspended in the air. Terri then added an airplane and directed it toward the baby. She spontaneously said, "It looks like it's gonna hit it!" Although I did not comment to Terri, it was noteworthy that this session marked a turning point in the treatment. Terri's anger and resentment toward the coming baby surfaced for the first time, indicating a shift in her defensive structure.

Terri's parents noted a decrease in her clinginess and an increase in her anger during this period. The anger was particularly strong at bedtime because Mrs. G. was no longer sleeping in Terri's room. This was accomplished as a result of hard work in conjoint biweekly parent counseling sessions. The news of her mom's pregnancy had clearly caused Terri a great deal of anxiety. This first emerged when Terri was at her father's house and he was sleeping with his girlfriend Kathy. It seemed that keeping Kathy away from dad, and mom away from her second husband, had been a way for Terri to manage her anxiety, fantasies, and feelings about what parents do in bed at night and her sexual concerns in general. Now that mom was no longer colluding with Terri's symptom and defense, Terri was able to express anger and other emotions.

Mr. and Mrs. G. responded very intuitively to Terri's anger and hostile behaviors and understood them as the child's first open admission that she had feelings about mother sleeping with stepfather and about the baby. Mr. and Mrs. G. used their sessions with me very productively to discuss helpful ways of addressing Terri's needs. Terri's natural father and his fiancée were also seen in periodic consultations for the same purpose. Simultaneously, the focus of Terri's sessions shifted to helping her discriminate between feelings and actions. As it became clearer that her thoughts and wishes could not hurt others, she was freer to express her feelings of fear about being displaced by the still unborn baby. Connections were made between being left alone at night and being left alone in general. By this time, Terri's anxiety symptoms had subsided.

Terri had been sleeping alone at night for several months by the time her brother was born (seven months into the treatment). She adjusted very well to his birth and was able to express both positive and negative emotions about him (e.g., he was "a pain" but at the same time "so cute"). With her parents' help Terri became involved in helping with the baby, yet both her mother and her stepfather made sure to spend time alone with her. One month after the birth of her brother, Terri requested family sessions to help her talk to her parents. Her parents welcomed this

request and used their biweekly sessions for this purpose. Weekly sessions of individual therapy with Terri
continued for three more months. During this time she
addressed changes in her household, peer relationships, and her frustration about never having time
with her father.

Termination

Terri became less resistant to treatment after we began
biweekly family sessions. She frequently mentioned
that having the evening alone with her mom and
stepfather made her feel as though she were once
again an only child. The pros and cons of being an only
child were explored and Terri spontaneously discussed
difficulties she experienced sharing mom with her
brother. Terri's parents worked on spending time with
her after the baby was put to bed and found ways to
involve her in helping with him so that Terri would not
feel excluded. Individual sessions were used to discuss
family sessions throughout this phase of treatment.

Approximately two months after beginning the
family sessions, Terri's parents commented that she
was "happy" and her "old self" again. This observation
and the conversation that followed prompted the family to explore Terri's readiness for ending treatment.
Using the developmental profile made it clear to me
that Terri's ego was functioning more efficiently. Her
defensive structure was significantly less rigid and she
showed a much more appropriate balance of affect
and defenses. Terri was able to self-soothe and had
become more resourceful in terms of finding alterna-

tive ways to satisfy her needs. Likewise, her parents reported that she coped with changes and challenges much better. The issue of ending treatment continued into a second family session and it was mutually decided that Terri was ready to stop treatment, allowing a four week period for saying goodbye.

During the first two termination sessions Terri did not address the fact that we would be stopping treatment. However, it was noteworthy that for the first time since she had started treatment she did not complain about having to come to her session. She used these sessions to play board games with me and simultaneously discussed school events, peer relationships, and the fact that she might be going to summer camp. There was a quality of connectedness and it seemed that Terri had come to trust me as someone she experienced as helpful.

The following week, during the third termination session, Terri wrote her father a letter in which she discussed her feelings of frustration about never seeing him. She wrote that she needed him to call her and to stay in touch more often and even alluded to the fact that she had been displaced by his fiancée Kathy. Interestingly, it was the awareness that Kathy was living with her dad that had brought about her symptoms ten months earlier. Terri and I were able to discuss how upsetting it was to miss dad so much. While Terri decided not to mail the letter, it somehow helped her to make sense of her inner experience. Remembering that she had drawn a girl mailing a letter during our first session, I asked Terri whether there was any connection, but she denied this. Nonetheless, I could not help wondering about the theme of wanting to say something or perhaps wanting to maintain a connection. I wondered whether a parallel process might be going on in terms of Terri feeling abandoned by me and perhaps wanting to stay in touch after the treatment ended. I broached this subject during our last session while Terri was drawing a picture of herself and her friends playing together. She denied feeling anything but happy about ending our sessions. Nonetheless, I did invite her to call, write, or have her mom call if she ever wanted to reconnect. This was communicated to Mr. and Mrs. G. as well and was deemed particularly important because of Terri's abandonment issues, which were apparently still present. She left the last session in a very casual manner and seemed unaffected by the fact that she would not be returning. However, I did note that Terri looked back before exiting the waiting room.

On a personal level, I had mixed feelings regarding ending treatment with Terri. On the one hand, I was struck by the strides she had made. She progressed from being an anxious, withdrawn child who drew smiling, "perfect" girls to becoming a child who was free and capable of acknowledging and clearly expressing frustration, anger, and needs. In addition, Terri was functioning at an age-appropriate level with regard to the latency-age tasks of achievement in academics and peer relations. However, despite these apparent gains I was concerned that we had not been able to address Terri's fantasies or feelings about what parents do in bed at night and her sexual concerns and anxieties in general. The fact that she was 10 years old and was already entering preadolescence when we ended treatment, made this a particularly strong concern. Moreover, because Terri's issues related to her dad were unresolved and she was still dealing with so many feelings, I questioned whether we had planned the termination prematurely. I experienced her goodbye as rather defensive in the sense that she could not acknowledge anything but happiness about leaving. This was complicated by the fact that Terri was approaching preadolescence at the time of termination.

In my experience this is the most difficult time to end therapy. Winnicott (1958) concurs, noting that latency is a particularly difficult time to stop treatment because of the many developmental changes brought about by the onset of preadolescence:

> How far during this period of relative calm in the instinctual world can the analyst claim to know the child? How far can the analyst deduce from what happens in such an analysis what the child was like at three or predict what the child will be like at thirteen? I am not sure of the answers to these questions but I know that I personally have been deceived, sometimes making a prognosis too favourable and sometimes not favourable enough. It is probably more easy to know what to do when the child is ill because then the obvious illness dominates the scene and treatment is not considered to be finished while the child's illness remains. [p. 123]

Perhaps these were some of the reasons why I questioned the completeness of Terri's treatment when we said goodbye and why, in fact, this is a common experience when ending treatment with latency-age youngsters. Terri's mom called me about eight months after termination to ask a question regarding her son, who was then just over a year old. Mrs. G. told me that Terri was happy and doing fine at home, at school, and in relation to her dad. I have not heard from the family since that time.

PART THREE

PREMATURE ENDINGS

Every child analyst's fear of failure concentrates on the worry that for one reason or another his young patient's treatment may come to an end prematurely.

Anna Freud

6

PREMATURE ENDINGS INITIATED BY PARENTS

In automobile terms, the child supplies the power but the parents have to do the steering.

Dr. Benjamin Spock

CHANGES IN LIFE CIRCUMSTANCES

Young families tend to move more frequently than do older, more settled ones. Job changes, divorce, remarriage, economic difficulties, a desire for better schools, and other factors lead young families to relocate and result in premature terminations when children are in treatment. When the child is moving away, leaving therapy constitutes just one of many real losses. Interpreting the child's play, verbalizations, and behavior as strictly transferential or related to leaving therapy would therefore minimize the many emotions and facets of change occurring in the child's life.

When ending treatment with children who are moving, the therapist must achieve three goals simultaneously. One goal is to help the child process and mourn the various losses that will result from the move. Depending on the extent of the move these losses may include neighborhood, school, teacher, classmates, community, and, on some level, the child's psychological sense of familiarity, predictibility, and security. In response to these losses some children may feel powerless, anxious, or angry. Therapy may be needed to address and work through these emotions. Another goal is to help the child prepare for the move by anticipating the changes that may occur. This will require meeting with parents to gather information about the new home, neighborhood, school, and so forth. Likewise, it is useful to work closely with parents to provide them with ideas that might foster the child's adjustment. In addition to helping the child work on issues pertaining to the move, it is, of course, important to address the ending of treatment and the meanings it has for the child. The therapist should help the child resolve feelings related to termination and should assess what services might be needed after the move. In cases where additional treatment is indicated, assistance with finding a therapist and transition planning is recommended.

Coppolillo (1988) notes that it is very important for the therapist to take an active stance when a child is going to be moving. He suggests that the therapist meet with the child's parents to ascertain the reasons for the move, find out how each family member perceives and feels about the move, and determine how much the child knows about the move:

The inevitability of the proposed move and the ways the parents propose to carry out the move should be weighed and examined in the context of the stage of treatment and the possible importance of the timing of the termination. The therapist may wish to agree with the parents' proposed termination date, or ask them to consider delaying it, or perhaps make it earlier. If, for example, the family must move on September 1st, and the therapist or the child were to have planned a vacation in July, the therapist may deem it wise to suggest that the termination date be set on the last session in June, rather than see the child for several sessions in August after a month's interruption. If an additional month or two is thought to be essential to the therapeutic gain, it is perfectly legitimate to ask the family to consider postponing a proposed relocation for that period. If a problem was sufficiently important to be treated, it is sufficiently important to be considered when the family is organizing their plans. To fail to do so may prejudice the decision to procure further help for the child in his new location, should he need it. [p. 318]

CASE ILLUSTRATION

Presenting Problem and Background

Andrew was 5½ years old when he was brought for treatment by his mother and stepfather. The presenting problems included poor social skills, bossiness with peers, a limited tolerance for frustration (which resulted in temper tantrums when things did not go his way), a tendency to blame others for difficulties, and separation anxiety. These behaviors and an overall sense of insecurity had increased since Andrew heard, six weeks earlier, that his teacher would be leaving because of her pregnancy.

Andrew's parents divorced when he was 2½ years old. He resided with his mother and older brother James and visited his dad every weekend for approximately eighteen months after the divorce. However, when Andrew was 4 his father moved out of state and their visits became significantly less frequent (usually once a month). That same year Andrew's mother remarried and quickly became pregnant. The baby, a boy who was named Robert, was born one month after Andrew started kindergarten. Treatment was sought three months later.

Prior to the birth of his baby brother, Andrew expressed concern to his mother about being "thrown away" after the baby was born. He became increasingly clingy, developed a fear of the dark, and frequently referred to himself as "dumb" or "stupid." Andrew would cry incessantly after leaving his mom to visit his dad and vice versa. After the baby's birth he became more bullyish. He was demanding and bossy with his classmates and would pinch his baby brother to make him cry.

Early and Middle Phases of Treatment

Andrew was seen for individual play therapy once a week and his mother and stepfather, Mr. and Mrs. J., were seen once or twice a month for parent counseling. In addition, regular telephone contact took place with Andrew's father. During the first play session, Andrew was accompanied by his mother and baby brother. Because he had extreme difficulty separating from his mother, she was invited to join us in the playroom. This provided Andrew with an emotional anchor while he explored the toys and became more comfortable. Interestingly, Andrew showed minimal interest in his mother during these sessions. In fact, it seemed that he was more interested in his brother. I recommended that Mrs. J. come alone with Andrew to the next session and he was able to separate without any difficulty. During this session Andrew revealed, while drawing a picture of his family, that he did not like when mom and Robert were alone for fear that he would "miss out on something."

Andrew was quite large in stature and his vocabulary was very sophisticated for a child his age. His mom was a counselor by training and had modeled a healthy awareness of feeling states, which made it comfortable for Andrew to share his feelings with me. He consistently used play sessions to show the therapist what he could do, how much he knew, how "good" he was at drawing or using art materials, and so forth. When playing board games he was extremely competitive and always had to be "better" and to win. During one session he took out the magic wand and I made believe I was a magic genie who could grant him three wishes. Andrew wished for "more time with dad," "more attention," and "more time with dad."

Andrew's strong wish for more time with his father was discussed during a parent session with his mom and stepfather. It was clear that Andrew missed his biological father and he was very open about this with everyone. However, this situation was complicated by the fact that Andrew's stepfather had been less available to him since Robert's birth. Mr. J. was able to discuss how Andrew's "rough and competitive" treatment of Robert also contributed to his emotional withdrawal from the boy. This theme was the focus of parent sessions, and as time went by Mr. J. developed much more effective strategies for dealing with Andrew's treatment of Robert.

As Andrew's teacher's departure approached, Andrew's separation anxiety increased. This was particularly true in relation to his biological father when weekend visits were coming to an end. Andrew adopted a tough exterior with peers and became even more competitive, always having to prove how much better he was. Apparently, the more insecure he felt the more rivalrous he became. I encouraged his parents (including the biological father) to focus on Andrew's positive behaviors and urged both fathers to spend some special time alone with Andrew. His teacher also planned a lunch alone with Andrew to emphasize how well he was doing and to discuss the new teacher who would be taking her place.

Andrew became quite attached to his younger brother in the weeks that followed. At about the same time, the family was trying to decide where Robert's crib should be placed now that he was outgrowing the bassinette. Their house had just three rooms, which meant that two of the boys would have to share a room. Andrew insisted that Robert share his room. During one session he explained that this would make

him feel "less lonely." Apparently, Andrew was beginning to see Robert as a companion. His parents reported that Andrew had become more nurturant and
helpful to Robert.

Termination Phase

Three and a half months into treatment, Andrew's
stepfather was offered a promotion out of state. Mr. J.'s
promotion came about quickly and the family had just
five weeks to prepare for the transition. Nonetheless,
this was a move that had been hoped for for several
reasons. It would bring Mrs. J. closer to her family of
origin and it would bring Andrew and his older brother
three hours closer to their dad. The latter was perceived as such a positive change for Andrew that it
overshadowed all other aspects of change involved in
the move. Nonetheless, Andrew's tendency to act in a
bullyish way when put in a situation that made him
feel vulnerable and fragile was a concern in view of the
fact that he would have to adjust to a new school, new
classmates, and the like. To address these issues, his
parents were seen more frequently during the month
prior to the move. These sessions focused on ways to
help Andrew make a smooth transition.

Andrew's initial reaction to the move was one of
excitement. However, as the move approached, he
became increasingly clingy with his mother. He began
to talk in a baby voice when his mother was "too busy"
attending to packing and other chores. Furthermore,
an increased incidence of lying became apparent. The
lying consistently involved blaming one or both broth-

ers for things that Andrew did wrong. In session, Andrew played with the doll house and there were frequent, unpredictable hurricanes, earthquakes, and eruptions. I pointed out his sense of how things change and how the people didn't have control. Andrew was unable to use this information and he was unable to work through his concerns and sense of powerlessness in the short period of time that we had together.

Because of the limited number of meetings Andew and I would have before the move, I decided to structure the last three sessions by introducing an art technique. I gave Andrew a coat of arms that he would cut out and decorate with "things that would help him when he moved" and "things he learned in therapy." This was my way of helping him process and prepare for the upcoming changes. Andrew was very amenable to this exercise, as he loved to draw. On the coat of arms he drew pictures representing "sharing," "smiling and saying hi" to make friends, and "talking to mom" when he gets sad, as well as a picture of himself and his dad.

In order to say goodbye, Andrew's parents managed to make the time to have a barbecue for neighbors and some of the classmates of both Andrew and his brother. Mr. J. had also taken pictures of the house where the family would be living, which helped to make it more real for the boys. I encouraged Mr. and Mrs. J. to take Andrew on a tour of the new school as soon as they arrived in their new town. With regard to Andrew's clinginess and lying, his parents were advised to focus on his underlying feelings of vulnerability and powerlessness. I recommended that Mr. and Mrs. J. involve Andrew in the move as much as possible by eliciting his help with packing or any other task related to the transition. This included talking to him about his new room, what color he would like to paint it, and so on.

My last session with Andrew followed his goodbye to classmates and teachers. He had just two days before the move and discussed how "millions" of boxes were in the house. Andrew was more in touch with the reality of the move. He brought the pictures of the new house with him to show me. Interestingly, he asked whether I would like to meet his older brother during this session. After doing so and saying goodbye to Andrew, I wondered whether his brother was a reassuring role model for him, someone who was going through the same changes, but, according to Mr. and Mrs. J., with significantly more confidence.

Andrew asked during one of our last sessions whether he could write to me the way he did to his teacher who had left. I of course responded with encouragement, but I have never heard from Andrew or his parents. They were given the phone number for the Psychological Association of the state to which they moved and were encouraged to call for a referral should Andrew need further assistance.

PARENT RESISTANCE

Nothing grows well in the shade of a big tree.
Constantin Brancusi

Termination of treatment with children is commonly initiated by changes in the child's life such as the start of a new school year, summer camp, moving away, financial constraints, insurance reimbursement issues, and the like. Weiss (1991) contends that these apparently external forces are often manifestations of underlying resistance in parents. He notes that parents often experience a reawakening of conflicts associated with their own childhood that parallel the issues and conflicts of their child's phase of development. The threat of undoing repression is therefore seen as the force that leads many parents to find reasons to interrupt treatment.

I would add that having a child in treatment can cause parents to experience anxiety or guilt (be it conscious or repressed) about their current or past parenting skills. Some parents become threatened by the relationship shared by the therapist and child and will end the treatment to be rid of the therapist who is perceived as a rival. Still other parents have such a strong identification with the child that they will tend to minimize the child's difficulties and resist further treatment. Perhaps the most difficult situation for therapists to deal with is when the parents terminate as a result of "giving up" or emotionally withdrawing from the child.

CASE ILLUSTRATION

Presenting Problem and Background

Carol, a child with severe separation anxiety, was previously described by this author (see Cangelosi 1995). She was 4 years old when her mother brought her for treatment. Carol's parents had separated seven months earlier and she had become increasingly clingy and frightened when separated from her mom. Every day Carol begged her mother not to leave for work and cried incessantly both before and after her mother departed. This occurred at bedtime as well.

Carol was an only child who had resided with her parents prior to their separation. However, because of extreme unhappiness in her marriage, Mrs. R. abruptly left her husband and moved back home with her parents, taking Carol out of state without Mr. R.'s consent. Carol lived with her mother and maternal grandparents throughout the treatment; she had minimal contact with her dad. He was extremely angry at his wife and would not call Carol in order to avoid speaking with Mrs. R. Likewise, Mrs. R. tended to minimize Carol's attachment to her dad. Her anger toward her husband prevented her from serving as a liaison so that Carol could maintain contact with him.

Mrs. R. reported that Carol often asked questions regarding her father, exhibited a lot of anger toward him, and often spoke of "hating" him. Mrs. R. suspected that this was her daughter's way of "acting tough" when in fact she was hurt. The mother believed that Carol "got this brave soldier routine" from her, as this had been her way of coping with stress and pain thoughout her life.

Early and Middle Phases of Treatment

Carol presented as an exceptionally appealing, albeit extremely serious child. She needed to have her mother in the room with us during the first two play therapy sessions and spent the entire first session exploring toys and showing them to her mom. She occasionally looked up at me but did not communicate directly with me until the second session. Despite the fact that her mom was also in the room during the second session, Carol asked me for assistance while building an airplane out of Fiddle Sticks. When she completed the structure she commented to her mother that she wished the plane could bring daddy. She then became agitated, took the plane apart, and said, "That's a make-believe plane, not a real one." From my perspective, this interchange showed how very difficult it was for Carol to even "play" with the idea of dad visiting. However, from Carol's mom's perspective this play scenario meant that treatment was "making Carol too upset." After the session Mrs. R. called to tell me that she was going to discontinue treatment for this reason. Education and support were provided; however, it was only after Mrs. R. spoke with her own counselor that her anxiety was alleviated and she could agree to further treatment.

By the third session Carol was able to come into the play room without her mother, provided that the door remained open so that she could see mother and physically reconnect when necessary. During this session, Carol lined up two rows of dinosaurs and explained that one row was following daddy and the other was following mommy. I commented that it must be hard for them to choose which one to follow. Carol then decided that the baby would have to ride on the mommy's back and went through great pains to make them "stay." After several unsuccessful attempts, she placed clay on the mother dinosaur's back and stuck the baby on top. Carol repeated this play theme several times in the weeks that followed. I commented on the baby's wish to ride on mom's back, addressing its fear, anxiety, and anger about being separate and alone.

Throughout this initial phase of treatment, Carol was able to play for short periods of time but became panicky when she realized she was alone (i.e., without her mom). She had to check in with her mother in the waiting room every few minutes. In contrast, by the third month of treatment she was able to stay in the therapy room without her mother and with the door closed. While she periodically wanted to show her mother something she made or to simply check in with her, Carol was clearly more comfortable with being separate. Her lack of worry and vigilance about mom's whereabouts resulted in an increased ability to become involved in imaginary play. Despite Carol's apparent progress, Mrs. R.'s resistance continued. In the third month of treatment she informed me that she had to cut back on parent counseling sessions because of financial difficulties. Although a fee adjustment was offered, she asked to come for parent counseling on an as-needed basis. With some encouragement she was able to commit to a minimum of one parent session every three weeks. Carol would continue her weekly sessions.

Major shifts took place in terms of Carol's separation anxiety during this phase of treatment. While she became increasingly tolerant of being away from mom for longer periods of time, she became more and more anxious, and at times intolerant, of separating from me. Initially, Carol became very angry at me at the end of sessions for "making her go." In the weeks that followed she developed a pattern of asking me, "Is it time to go?" from five minutes into the session until it was in fact time to leave. Play themes shifted as well. During one session she developed a scenario in which a baby doll was crying and the mother was "too tired to hold the baby" but the baby was able to seek comfort from the father. Interestingly, it was during this time that Carol's mother was planning a trip to take her to see her dad and to see whether there was any possibility for a reconciliation.

It was clear by this point in treatment that Carol felt safe enough to wish for a comforting father and had the freedom to play without having to remind herself that it was "only make believe" as she had done with the airplane previously. This session seemed to be Carol's way of preparing for her visit with dad. There also seemed to be a transferential meaning to Carol's play, because it paralleled the increased comfort she was experiencing with me. Carol was beginning to internalize the idea of being able to attain comfort from other sources when mother was not available.

Carol returned from visiting her father with a smile! It was the first time I had seen her smile in the four months that we had been working together. During this session she played peek-a-boo with me. Each time she jumped out, I acted surprised and made statements reflecting the theme of disappearance and reappearance (e.g., "Just when I think I'm alone, I realize you're still there" and vice versa). Later in this session, Carol asked whether I still had the clay family figures that she had made and that I had promised to keep for her. I reminded Carol that her basket of toys was still in her special place even though we had been separated for a few weeks. Interestingly, Carol did not play with the figures after finding them. But she was clearly relieved to see that she still had a place with me and had not been forgotten.

In the weeks that followed, Carol played house and repeatedly staged a nighttime routine with the baby doll that included feeding, changing, and then laying the baby down to sleep, telling it to go to sleep while shutting the lights off. Carol would then lie down herself and instruct me to "go to sleep." She was clearly attempting to master her fear of the dark and her struggles with bedtime. According to her mom, bedtime was still a difficult time despite the fact that Carol had become significantly more comfortable with separating from mom during the day.

Termination Phase

Two weeks after returning from her visit with Carol's father (four and a half months into the treatment), Mrs. R. called and left a message on my answering machine informing me that she had decided to pursue a divorce from Carol's father. She also informed me that she had decided to terminate treatment so that she could save money for an apartment. She thanked me for my help and noted that Carol was doing much better. I called Mrs. R. back, but she was not open to discussing the possibility of a fee adjustment and was set on terminating the treatment. When I alerted her that terminating so abruptly might be upsetting to Carol in light of her history, difficulties with separation, and attachment to me, Mrs. R. agreed to come in for one last session so that Carol could have the opportunity to say goodbye.

During the last session Carol became closed and angry when I attempted to talk about saying goodbye. She played with the baby doll and repeatedly told it not to cry while she (the mother) got ready to go to work. Throughout this session Carol seemed extremely anxious. She walked in and out of the room and in and out of the toy closet and repeatedly started sentences and "forgot" what she was going to say. In an attempt to make the therapy real (and not something that disappears), I gave Carol the clay figures that she had made during the initial phase of treatment. Mrs. R. was asked to join us during the last few minutes of the session so that we could all say goodbye.

Processes Underlying Mrs. R.'s Decision to Terminate

Throughout Carol's treatment, attempts were made to educate and involve her parents in the therapeutic process. While Mr. R. approved of his daughter's treatment, he did not take part in the therapy because of his physical distance and his related sense of being an outsider and helpless regarding Carol's fate. Although Mrs. R. sought treatment, she was very anxious that therapy would create further difficulties and label Carol "problemed." Furthermore, Mrs. R. was continually attempting to ward off guilt about being responsible for her daughter's difficulties. To come to treatment was, for her, to admit that something was wrong and presumably that she was the cause.

Mrs. R. struggled with her anger toward Carol's father and her concern that it might not be in Carol's best interest to be so far away from him. Unfortunately, when these thoughts surfaced she defended against them by totally denying her husband's significance to Carol. The more I attempted to address these issues in the parent counseling sessions, the more she withdrew from treatment and the more fearful she became that Carol's treatment would somehow hurt her. In this respect, Mrs. R. was overidentified with Carol. That is, the more anxious the treatment made her, the more she presumed that it was also increasing Carol's anxiety.

Mrs. R. was clearly too frightened to address her own internal conflicts, which seemed to resonate with what Carol was experiencing. I suspected that she also felt separation anxiety both in relation to her own family of origin and in relation to Carol. Mrs. R. had developed a "brave little soldier routine" to deal with her anxiety and vulnerability. This contributed to her ending Carol's treatment so abruptly. Unfortunately, Carol's repeated message to the doll during her last session ("Don't cry") reveals that she was in fact attempting to be a brave soldier as well.

While I was not able to change the course of events that took place in terms of the premature termination, insisting on at least one session to say goodbye did carry an important message. During our last meeting, I made sure to convey to both Carol and her mom that they were both much too important to simply flee and vanish without a goodbye. I also gave Carol a souvenir of our work together (the clay family) to make it real and something that she could take with her in a concrete way. Both Carol and Mrs. R. were also given a very clear message that I would be available should they want or need to return at a later date. Interestingly, Mrs. R. took me up on this offer and called three and a half years later when Carol was struggling with issues related to her father's remarriage.

7

PREMATURE
ENDINGS INITIATED
BY THE CHILD

The plant would like to grow
And yet be embryo;
Increase, and yet escape
The doom of taking shape.
                    Richard Wilbur

CLINICAL CONSIDERATIONS

It is a common experience for child therapists to be informed that their young patients wish to discontinue treatment. The abrupt and often unpredictable manner with which this news is often conveyed makes it a particularly difficult situation to deal with. The child's wish to end psychotherapy can be brought about by a number of factors. For instance, children can become resistant to further treatment when anxiety-provoking or emotionally charged issues surface; when regressive pulls occur; when parents are ambivalent, resistant or threatened by treatment; or when an attachment to the therapist takes place. With regard to the latter, some children begin to feel disloyal to their parents or vulnerable due to previous disappointments with attachment figures.

It is not uncommon for children to express a desire to stop treatment when they sense that their parent(s) want to end treatment. This can be a response to loyalty conflicts or a wish to control the ending themselves. The desire to discontinue treatment can also stem from a thrust toward further development. In some cases it may suggest that the child is "back on track" developmentally and no longer in need of treatment. However, even when this is true, a period of working through is important. Anna Freud has pointed out that even after an agreed termination there should not be an abrupt ending of contact but a more gradual detaching process. This might be done by scheduling sessions less frequently or by setting up a follow up session after a vacation or summer/holiday break.

In some situations, a child's expression that s/he wants to stop treatment does not necessarily mean that the child truly wishes to terminate. Instead, it may reflect a fear of being abandoned or rejected (Sandler et al. 1980). The need to understand latent meanings of the child's wish and to work through these responses is an important part of the termination process. When a child expresses a wish to stop treatment I ask myself a series of questions. These might include: Where is the child in terms of his/her development? Is the child ready to try things out without treatment? Would ending provoke a thrust toward development? Is the child attempting to avoid anxiety-provoking material? Is s/he becoming too attached to me and (a) experiencing loyalty conflicts or (b) attempting to control the process of saying goodbye? What message is the parent conveying to the child regarding treatment and its ending? What kinds of experiences has the child had with loss/separation and what messages need to be worked through in this regard? A rule of thumb with all terminations is to not collude with the child's or the parents' resistance when it comes to addressing issues of loss.

CASE ILLUSTRATION

Presenting Problem and Background

Brian was 6 years old when his mother brought him for treatment. The presenting problems included extreme separation difficulties, aggressiveness, fighting with other children, and school avoidance. Brian's remark that he would "rather die than to go to school" initiated Mrs. K.'s phone call to me.

Brian's parents had separated when he was 2½ years old. He had two siblings, an older brother of 8 and a younger sister of 4½. The children lived with their mother and visited with their father one day a week. Mrs. K. reported that the marriage had ended because Brian's dad was an alcoholic who had been physically and emotionally abusive toward her. Although he never hit the children, they were reportedly frightened of him. The separation was initiated by an order of protection that Mrs. K. obtained following an argument in which Mr. K. threatened to kill her. This

exacerbated the already tumultuous relationship between Brian's parents. Despite their separation the
intense conflict continued to the extent that it took
them four years to agree on a divorce settlement. The
divorce was finalized eight months prior to the start of
Brian's treatment.

Mrs. K. noted that Brian's difficulties with separation and his school avoidance began a month or so
after the divorce was finalized. He also became more
aggressive at that time. When I inquired about changes
in the home that might account for these symptoms,
Mrs. K. replied that Brian's father had pulled away
from the children since the divorce and that she had
become more verbal about her negative feelings about
his father. Mrs. K. went on to say that she felt very
overwhelmed by her full-time job and the demands of
raising three young children alone. She openly expressed resentment and hostility toward her ex-
husband for putting her in this situation. Mrs. K. felt
guilt about losing her temper with the children when
they were uncooperative, and she reported that Brian
often got the brunt of this because of his aggressiveness. When Brian was uncooperative or bullyish toward his siblings she frequently accused him of being
"just like his father."

At the time of intake it was apparent that Mrs. K.
could benefit from treatment for herself but she was
not open to this. Nonetheless, she did agree to meet for
parent counseling and gave me permission to work
with Brian's dad, warning me that he would probably
not care enough to be involved. She informed me that
Brian's older brother had been in counseling for over a

year and his dad did not participate in that treatment.

Contrary to Mrs. K.'s prediction, Brian's father willingly came to meet with me. He presented as a calm and rather stoic man who described Brian in much the same way as did Mrs. K. Interestingly, Mr. K. thanked me for including him in the intake and said that he had felt like an outsider with the children ever since the separation four years earlier. Mr. K. reported that he did not want the divorce and openly admitted to drinking and losing his temper at his wife when they were married. He attributed these behaviors to her nagging him and putting him down and noted that she did the same with Brian and his older brother. Mr. K. expressed concern that Mrs. K. "bad-mouthed me to everyone including the kids." He had apparently adopted a passive, uninvolved stance in relation to the children because of his conviction that they needed their mom more than their dad at such a young age. In view of his affect and passive, resigned stance I questioned whether he was suffering from depression, but he denied this. Like his ex-wife, Mr. K. was not interested in a referral for treatment for himself but was willing to see me for parent counseling as part of Brian's treatment.

Early and Middle Phases of Treatment

As I approached the waiting room to greet Brian for his first session, I heard him say, "You better sit by me" to his mother. The tone of his voice was demanding and rather aggressive. In contrast, he related to me in a polite, timid, and soft-spoken manner. This polarity intensified as the session progressed. Brian used the entire first session to ask me questions about how toys and games worked, and in each instance he demanded that his mother "make" them work. His speech and movements were characterized by anxious speed and he flitted from one toy to another.

During this session Brian asked to use the bathroom and demanded that his mother go with him. When I inquired about this, Mrs. K. explained that Brian "needed help wiping himself." The fact that Brian was having such a difficulty was striking, but what was even more surprising was the dispassionate manner with which Mrs. K. related this information. When she and Brian returned to the play room Brian's level of aggression, anxiety, and anger escalated. He took out toy soldiers and pretended to shoot his mother. He then began to poke her with the guns. The more she tolerated, the more Brian escalated. Eventually he began to throw the soldiers at her, but she still did not set limits. At this point I told Brian that he would not be allowed to hurt himself or anyone else in the play room. He seemed surprised by my intervention but nonetheless cooperated.

Brian's sense of needing his mother's help, and his related lack of trust in his ability to do things for and by himself, emerged as a major issue in the weeks that followed. Although he was able to tolerate having his mother sit in the waiting room (with the door half closed) by the second session, he repeatedly demanded that she escort him to the bathroom for several weeks in order to wipe him. By that time, I had had a chance to meet with Mrs. K. individually to discuss a plan for addressing this behavior. During our fourth session, when Brian got up to use the bathroom and began to yell for his mother I told him that this time he should wipe himself the way his mom did. He insisted that he needed his mother's help; with encouragement, however, he went to the bathroom alone. Brian repeatedly called to his mother in protest, but with support from me she was able to serve as a cheerleader for Brian from outside the bathroom door.

When Brian returned from the bathroom he seemed cheerful and no mention was made of the bathroom incident. Yet it was interesting to note that he adopted a rather helpless stance when he returned to the playroom. He repeatedly attempted to elicit my aid in assembling the toy soldiers before even trying to do so himself. This tendency increased in the weeks that followed. It appeared that the more autonomous Brian became, the more he feared losing his mom, and in the transference, me. This issue was worked on by means of encouragement in the playroom and helping Mrs. K. to learn ways of assisting Brian through emotional support instead of doing things for him.

Brian played out repetitive war themes in the opening phase of treatment. Each week he arranged the army soldiers differently and struggled to decide who were the "good guys" and who were the "bad guys." During one session this play caused Brian to regress. He began to talk like a baby and repeatedly said "good guy, bad guy, good guy, bad guy" while banging the heads of two soldiers together. The most obvious metaphor revealed in this play was Brian's anxiety about his parents' being at war and his desire to make sense of who was good or right. At a deeper level, Brian seemed to be attempting to find something safe to hold onto. If one parent was good, then perhaps that would provide a sense of safety and security. The fact that neither parent was all good seemed to surface during this session. At yet another level, I believe Brian was attempting to integrate a sense of who he was (i.e., good or bad).

Brian had interpreted his mom's accusations that he was like his father as meaning that he was bad and could also be "divorced." His regressed, dependent behaviors were a compromise formation that enabled him to keep his mom close and lessen the fear and anxiety of being cast away as he perceived his dad to have been. However, this did not seem to work. Each time Mrs. K. gave in to Brian's regressed behaviors, as when she wiped him, his anxiety was aroused by the blurring of the mother–son boundary. This experience exacerbated Brian's oedipal feelings, which were already enormous given his history of having kept his mother during the oedipal phase when his father was forced to leave. Brian was overwhelmed with fear of retaliation from his father, fear that was likely exacerbated by his having seen his father abuse his mother when he, Brian, was at the height of the oedipal conflict.

During the third and fourth months of treatment Brian's play themes revolved around cops and robbers. Each week he would be a cop and I was instructed to be a robber who had just been put in jail. Brian would pretend to be sleeping and would instruct me to sneak out of jail. Repeatedly, I would be caught and Brian, the cop, would scold me and remind me that I could not "get away with it." He then would become passive and somewhat apologetic and would attempt to undo the aggressive stance he had taken. This play theme appeared to be a metaphor for Brian's superego, which was being gradually neutralized. The repetitive play was a vehicle through which Brian was working through and mastering oedipal issues and more specifically his confused identification with his father.

During this phase of the treatment, Brian's attachment to me became more and more intense and he evinced increasing levels of anxiety at the end of each session. He would cry and at times even refuse to leave despite the fact that I provided him with several reminders when the end of the session was approaching. Simultaneously, Mrs. K. reported that Brian was separating from her more easily and was happier and less demanding at home. During our fifteenth sesion, I gave Brian a plastic bin in which he could keep several toys. The bin was kept in a special place in the office where it would remain safe and untouched until our next session. This was done to provide Brian with an anchor or sense of belonging that would, I hoped, alleviate his anxiety about separating. Despite his positive reaction to this idea, Brian had so much difficulty leaving this session that his mother eventually had to carry him out of the office. Brian then refused to return the following week, and his mother was unfortunately not able to take charge and get him to our session.

The following week Brian reported that he missed me during our break and told me that he wished I were his mother. He also informed me that his father had gone away on vacation the week before, and he complained that he never got to go along with him. Brian again had a very hard time leaving the session. Several days later Mrs. K. called to tell me that Brian did not wish to continue treatment and stated that it was becoming too hard for her to get him to leave the sessions. I sensed that taking charge, as she was forced to do to induce him to leave, was causing her much anxiety and I empathized with this while simultaneously attempting to educate her about the importance of continuing Brian's treatment.

Mrs. K. and I discussed the fact that Brian was upset about his father's departure. I believed that Brian was acting out his feelings with me in the transference. The endings of our sessions, which were already experienced as anxiety-provoking and perhaps rejecting, were causing Brian's feelings about his father's departure to surface. His refusal to return to treatment seemed to be his way of turning the table and becoming the rejector or the person in charge instead of the passive person being left. Parenthetically, this appeared to be another way in which Brian was trying to work out his confused feelings related to identifying with his dad.

Prior to Brian's next session, Mrs. K. came in for a parent counseling session to discuss ways to address Brian's resistance. At that time she agreed that it was important to continue Brian's treatment so that he could work through his many conflicts.

Termination Phase

Mrs. K. informed me at the beginning of the next session that Brian had given her a very hard time about coming. She told me that it would be Brian's last session for the time being because of his resistance about attending and about leaving. Unfortunately, this was a closed subject! During the session Brian played with the doll house and created a fire scene that seemed to be a metaphor for the exaggerated degree of power he had in the family as well as for his sense of not being taken care of by his parents. The mother doll cried helplessly in the bedroom, holding a baby. The father was not strong enough to get in to rescue them until the little boy came to help. The boy proceeded to knock the door down while yelling, "You're weak" to the father. Brian moved quickly from this scene to repetitive cop and robber scenes that we played for the remainder of the session. He cried intensely when it was time to leave and I reassured him that he could return at any point if he'd like. Despite several followup phone calls to both Mr. and Mrs. K. they were not willing to continue individual treatment for Brian or parent counseling for themselves.

Processes Underlying Brian's Resistance to Treatment

Brian's resistance to treatment began to emerge as a result of his difficulty in separating from me. Given his history of separation anxiety, this was partly transferential, a result of unresolved rapprochement issues.

However, it seemed that as Brian's attachment to me as a real object grew, he became extremely vulnerable. This was partly due to previous disappointments with his parents, who had been unable to provide him with a sense of security.

The fact that I did provide a safe environment for Brian caused him to wish that I were his mother. This fantasy was threatening in and of itself, but its oedipal implications were too much for Brian's fragile ego to deal with. Nonetheless, his treatment would not have ended at such a crucial time, and particularly in such an abrupt manner, had one or both parents been able to support that part of Brian's ego that liked and benefited from treatment. It appeared that Mrs. K. colluded with Brian's resistance instead of encouraging him to work through it. Clearly, this was partly due to her tendency to give in to Brian's wishes and demands as opposed to setting limits and providing structure. I've also wondered how she was affected by Brian's display of emotion toward me and whether this did not threaten her to the extent that she too needed to stop the treatment so abruptly. This would certainly explain why she decided not to return for parent counseling even though Brian was unable to continue his treatment. Unfortunately, Mr. K.'s tendency to retreat passively was recapitulated when he too discontinued parent counseling.

8

PREMATURE ENDINGS INITIATED BY THE THERAPIST

When you have
once had
a great joy
it lasts always
quivers gently
on the edge of all the
insecure adult days
subdues inherited dread
makes sleep deeper.
                    Tove Ditlevsen

CLINICAL CONSIDERATIONS

Some therapist-initiated terminations occur because of countertransference. For the purpose of this book, I would like to borrow Weiss's (1991) definition of countertransference as "the various reactions the analyst has that interfere with the orderly termination of the child's analysis." Weiss notes that "such reactions may involve supporting or even initiating a premature termination; or they may support the child's and/or the parent's wish not to [address issues related to the desire to] terminate. They may involve the analyst's inability to face the various affects that are provoked by the termination process and/or his helping the child avoid facing these affects" (p. 270). In accordance with this definition, it is clearly of the utmost importance that therapists undertake self analysis whenever they make a decision regarding ending or not ending treatment with children. This includes instances when they agree or disagree with the child's or parent's decision to terminate treatment or when they themselves initiate termination.

On occasion the therapist will initiate termination because of changes in his or her life circumstances. Such changes might include illness, a new job, relocation, or pregnancy. Terminating treatment under these conditions leaves the therapist with two kinds of challenges. The first has to do with the tasks inherent in all terminations and the second involves examination of transference and countertransference reactions stemming from the fact that termination is occurring for a reason that is not related to the treatment.

Clearly, all terminations, even those that are planned following successful treatment, evoke emotions, conflicts, and defensive reactions in child patients, their parents, and their therapists. Even in the most ideal terminations, we as therapists are confronted with our own past separations. Issues related to separation and individuation, dependency, autonomy, abandonment, and loss may be reawakened, or may emerge in new, previously unknown forms, when ending treatment with children. Likewise, our personal needs, sense of professional competence, and attachment to specific children may bring about emotional responses at the time of termination. When termination is planned because of the child's progress, these matters can be explored and worked through while we simultaneously help the child (and the parents) to resolve their own issues pertaining to termination. However, a number of additional difficulties complicate this process when termination is prompted by changes in the therapist's life.

Dewald (1980) notes that, for the patient, therapist-initiated termination "represents a unilateral decision made by someone else—a decision which does not take into account his or her own emotional or therapeutic needs. It may be perceived as a repetition of arbitrary, unexpected and 'selfish' behavior of earlier key figures particularly when there have been significant or traumatic separations earlier in the patient's life" (p. 14). Dewald stresses that the patient's affective and defensive response will usually be consistent with reactions to similar previous situations.

For the therapist, self-initiated termination can bring about a number of personal reactions. Feelings of guilt, frustration (for leaving before the "end"), sadness, and depression are not uncommon. Likewise, stress resulting from the upcoming life change can cause avoidance, lack of focus, decathexis, emotional withdrawal, and eagerness to be done with professional obligations. Therapists' feelings of guilt may make them reluctant to offer comments or interpretations and may result in decreased tolerance for the child's anger or negative reactions. Therapists may also minimize their importance to the child and may collude with the child to avoid sadness or loss reactions. They may delay informing the child about the impending termination or may arrange for immediate transfer to a new therapist to reduce guilt and avoid painful transference and countertransference reactions (Dewald 1980).

With regard to transferring cases, Anna Freud states that "transfer should be considered as an alternative to complete termination, and it should be decided whether the patient's condition warrants such transfer. It is generally advisable for a patient who must terminate with one therapist to wait and only later start again with another therapist if necessary" (Sandler et al. 1980, p. 246). While this approach may not be indicated for all children, it highlights the importance of not "replacing" the departing therapist before the child has the opportunity to work through the loss. Therapists who are forced to leave patients are not always clear about the progress that the child has made and may tend to underestimate their role and their therapeutic effectiveness as they seek a replacement to ensure that the child is taken care of (Dewald 1980).

PREGNANCY

Literature addressing the impact of the therapist's pregnancy suggests that the anticipated absence due to maternity leave is as significant for the child as is the fact of the pregnancy itself (Miller 1992). Pregnancy can accelerate the pace of treatment, as it tends to facilitate the unfolding of central issues experienced by the child (Fenster et al. 1986, Guy et al. 1986, Miller 1992). Miller highlights this point in her description of David, a 4½-year-old child who presented with an oppositional disorder. This child's use of oppositional behavior did not surface in the therapeutic relationship until he began to address termination issues related to the therapist's pregnancy. Thus termination served to trigger David's underlying sense of powerlessness, anger, and sadness.

During the six week termination phase, Miller used a calendar to point out the number of remaining sessions for David. He initially participated in this activity but later withdrew and refused to look at the calendar. As the termination phase progressed, David became increasingly agitated and oppositional at the end of sessions. He refused to clean up toys and hid in order to prolong the sessions. When Miller reflected David's feelings and desire to control the ending process, he calmed down and become more cooperative. However, on two occasions, she chose to carry David out of the room in order to enforce the therapeutic time frame. This intervention seemed to have a positive effect as David then left willingly and demonstrated no further difficulties. Miller notes, however, that David covered his ears and said "Stop talking!" whenever she offered any interpretation of abandonment issues triggered by the ending of treatment.

Miller candidly discusses how distressing David's oppositional and disorganized behaviors were for her. She describes feeling unprepared for his regression and experienced it as a negation of the therapeutic progress that had taken place. In addition, Miller's empathy toward David caused her to experience herself as he saw her—"a cruel, abandoning person" (p. 632). She writes:

> The David-attuned part of me felt terrified and angry, but I was only minimally aware of these feelings. More

often I felt guilt because I unknowingly believed I was cruel and abandoning; I was unable to examine the source of this belief or to realize that cruel and abandoning was how David saw me, not how I truly was. I coped with my resultant guilt and shaky self-esteem by questioning the value of my therapeutic work with him. My guilt and doubts served to distance me from David, thereby providing some relief from my distress and allowing me to approach sessions with some emotional detachment. I was unable to realize that I needed to choose to detach and think through whose distress belonged to whom. Such a conscious process would have enabled me to remember that the shift in our relationship actually allowed me greater access to David's core issues and defenses. [p. 632]

Miller notes that although a return to work was planned after her six-week maternity leave, some children were unable to use this information to mitigate the sadness, sense of abandonment, fears, and anger stirred up by her leaving: an absence that extended for six weeks was simply incomprehensible for these children.

Dr. Tamara Shulman, an analyst and respected colleague who has taken two maternity leaves from her private practice, was interviewed for some insights regarding termination issues related to pregnancy (Shulman 1996). She noted that the most pervasive theme among child patients was their wish to be called after the baby was born. For many children this reflected a need to know that she was still interested in them. Children with histories of traumatic separations that had led them to associate hospitals with danger needed to know that she was all right. Still other children needed to feel involved. Some even made drawings for the hospital or the baby's room.

Many child patients developed an identification with the unborn baby that manifested in a desire for the baby to be the same sex as themselves or in an insistence that this was the case. One little boy was so sure that the baby was a boy that he claimed his doctor had told him so. Similarly, a set of twins insisted that Shulman would be having twins. Many children expressed curiosity about the name that would be chosen for the baby. This seemed to reflect the underlying question: "Do you want a child like me?" Shulman noted that, although some children could have ended treatment prior to or at the time of her maternity leave, many children and parents chose not to. They needed to come back when she returned from her leave so that they could say goodbye on their own terms.

RELOCATION: CASE ILLUSTRATION

Presenting Problem and Background

Ronny was seen in individual play therapy for approximately sixteen months, when I informed him that I would be moving out of state. An only child, Ronny was 8 years, 3 months old when his parents sought treatment to "help him with his feelings."

The developmental history revealed that in kindergarten Ronny had demonstrated difficulties with his attention span and a hearing problem had been diagnosed. He underwent surgery to remedy the problem. However, shortly after the surgery, Ronny developed social and behavioral problems at home and at school. He did not follow directions, would not respond to limits unless consequences were defined, and exhibited poor social skills. In the classroom he would grab things from others, interrupt others when he thought they were doing something incorrectly, and so forth. His peers came to see Ronny as "different" and ostracized him because he was overweight.

Ronny was in the early part of the second grade at the time of the initial intake. He was reportedly doing better in school because his teacher was "warm yet structured." Nonetheless, he struggled with homework and would get butterflies in his stomach on Monday mornings. Psychological testing revealed superior intelligence. However, there were numerous indications of distractibility and anxiety. Ronny's home life was described as extremely stressful due to the fact that both parents maintained high-level corporate positions and Ronny's dad was often unavailable.

Approximately two months prior to the intake, Ronny began to experience nightmares that caused him to wake up screaming several times each night. He was fearful by night because of these nightmares and fearful by day because he was being ostracized by his peers. According to his parents, Ronny had no friends and no special interests or hobbies. He had recently told his mother, "Life isn't fair to me," after several peers made fun of him. This incident prompted his parents to seek therapy.

Early and Middle Phases of Treatment

Ronny arrived for his first session with much enthusiasm. He separated from his mother easily and began the session by stating that he knew I was a "feeling doctor" who could help him with his "sadness." He proceeded to tell me that he had been sad because his peers made fun of him and called him fat. Ronny spontaneously described several situations with peers that revealed that he had handled social situations in a provocative manner. His stories also made it clear that he had difficulty sharing, taking turns, and compromising. He conveyed a sense of loneliness and a related anxiety about not fitting in with his peers.

Ronny presented as a very sensitive, somewhat sad boy who was keenly aware of feeling lonely, "different," and like an outsider in relation to his agemates. He was a very appealing child with a warm and engaging manner. However, it was quite striking that he did not smile at all throughout the first few months of treatment. His seriousness, combined with his large stature, weight, outstanding verbal ability, and precocious level of awareness made Ronny appear older than his age. His speech tended to be pressured and he was extremely fidgety. He had such difficulty sitting still that he would spontaneously rise while talking and begin to pace about the room. This seemed to happen most frequently when he was talking about upsetting experiences.

It was noteworthy that Ronny chose to talk instead of exploring the toys and games throughout the first two months of treatment. He enjoyed the one-to-one contact and used the sessions to discuss ongoing problems with peers as well as interesting things that he was learning in school. Ronny arrived for our eighth session very excited about a science experiment he had done and asked whether he could draw a diagram of it for me. While he drew the diagram, I asked questions so that Ronny could hear himself verbalize what he had learned. He had little awareness of how bright and talented he was; my questions and enthusiasm were intended to provide him with some of the esteem and pride that he was clearly lacking. It was interesting to note that Ronny's speech was not at all pressured during this session, nor did he need to fidget or pace. It appeared that the drawing served the same function as the pacing, namely to discharge energy.

Ronny became much more animated during our subsequent sessions and began to smile more as the months went by. He frequently drew pictures of places he had been, ideas he had, and, from time to time, "monsters in [his] head." Ronny also chose to play with cards or board games, or to do interactive drawing (such as the squiggle game) during his sessions. Game play provided ample opportunity for me to model cooperation, sharing, and taking turns. Ronny caught on quickly and demonstrated no problems in these areas when playing games with me. Likewise, his parents reported that he got along fine with girls in his class. Ronny's social difficulties became centered around boys, whom he experienced as "bullies."

My montly meetings with Ronny's parents stressed family dynamics as well as his need for recreational and social activities. Four months into treatment, his mother signed Ronny up for a swimming class, which he loved. The class challenged him because he did not have a good sense of body awareness and tended to be clumsy. It also helped him to lose weight and become more confident and playful. Ronny talked openly and enthusiastically about his swim class, using therapy to process goals, accomplishments, and disappointments.

With regard to his distractibility in the classroom, I encouraged Ronny's mom to ask for assistance from the Child Study Team. The school psychologist developed a behavioral program with Ronny's teacher that stressed paying attention, not calling out, and waiting his turn. Interestingly, helping his teacher pass papers, water plants, and the like proved to be effective rewards. I kept in contact with the school to monitor Ronny's progress and needs.

That summer Ronny went to a day camp for boys and had the opportunity to try out many new recreational and social skills. This was an excellent opportunity for him to overcome his fears and anxieties. One of the themes of his treatment revolved around "bullies" and how to deal with them. At one point, he wanted to quit camp because older boys had been throwing rocks at him and calling him names. Ronny's aggression tended to be turned inward and he adopted a passive approach to such situations. He was overidentified with females, since his father was emotionally absent and his house was run by his mother. Despite these obstacles, Ronny was able to explore options other than quitting camp and was able to confront the bullies with the help of his camp counselors. As he became more assertive, Ronny's nightmares became significantly less frequent.

Ronny started to take karate lessons three months before I informed him that I would be moving out of state. The classes were clearly helping him become more focused, confident, assertive, and disciplined.

Termination Phase

I informed Mrs. J. of my impending move during our monthly parent-counseling session, and we discussed the importance of the final phase of treatment. She agreed to a six-week termination period that would focus on helping Ronny to consolidate his gains, to prepare for the upcoming school year (we ended in late July), and to say goodbye. During the ending phase, Mrs. J. and I discussed the many strides that Ronny had made since beginning treatment. I also outlined my concerns about his need for improvement in social skills and self-confidence, and about issues related to his feeling lonely and different. We agreed that Ronny could wait before seeing a new therapist, but that it would be important for her to keep a close eye on the child, especially at the start of the new school year. Also highlighted was the unresolved issue of Ronny's feelings about his dad's lack of availability.

I informed Ronny of my move at the beginning of our next session. He began to ask lots of questions about where I would be going and what I would be doing. On the surface, Ronny seemed excited about the news and spoke of how his kindergarten teacher had also moved away. But there was a lot going on below the surface! Later in this session, Ronny took out a felt board and created a scene in which a boat with one young bear was drifting down a stream, leaving behind another bear. Ronny's play was strikingly different during this session compared to what I observed in any previous or subsequent hours. He played in a much more solitary, somber manner, making me acutely aware of his sadness and my own. I had known that it would be difficult to say goodbye to the patients I was working with, but I wasn't aware until this session how guilty, sad, and conflicted I was about letting go. This was particularly true with Ronny, as I had grown very fond of him and was touched by the many struggles he worked out in his treatment. At an intuitive level I felt that interpreting Ronny's play would somehow take away from his working-through process. I chose to respect his need for emotional distance. Thus no words were spoken about the boat scenario by either Ronny or myself. When he completed it, he put the felt board back in the box with the scene remaining. This was unusual for Ronny, as he had typically taken scenes apart when working with such toys. I noted that Ronny wanted somehow to keep the picture as a remembrance. He proceeded to play Jenga with me, a game that allowed for relating, connecting, and cooperation. Ronny became animated during this part of the session, and I emphasized the theme of "working together." (Parenthetically, it was Ronny's felt-board scene that served as the impetus for this book!)

When he returned the following week, Ronny asked to play the squiggle game, another connecting and relating enterprise. From each of five squiggles

Ronny drew in this order: a question mark, a rattle-snake, a plane discharging smoke, a palm tree, and a rattlesnake on the screen of a television with a remote control on the side. I believe that the first drawing, the question mark, depicted Ronny's uncertainty about the future without treatment. As the game progressed, he expressed his anxiety about his impulses and his fearfulness via the rattlesnake (a theme in his night-mares). He demonstrated the ability to discharge anxi-ety and impulses through the sublimation represented by the airplane. The palm tree depicted the calmness as well as Ronny's focus on the future (an upcoming trip to Florida with his parents). Finally, the rattle-snake on the television screen, drawn exactly like the previous rattlesnake, served to reassure him that he indeed had the capacity to contain his impulses and to achieve distance from and control over his fears. Ronny left the session in an animated fashion.

The following week, he chose to play Jenga and Don't Break the Ice. While playing, he told me that he thought he would be okay when we stopped our meetings. However, he told me that he sometimes got scared that the kids at school would make fun of him in the third grade. He recalled "how hard life used to be" and described vivid memories of peers mocking and rejecting him. In addition to processing these painful experiences, Ronny and I worked, throughout the termination process, to identify specific behaviors and attitudes that had caused positive changes in his life. Ronny internalized and took ownership of these abilities to such an extent that he insisted on trying things out without a new counselor. I was concerned that he might have been rejecting a new therapist because of feelings of abandonment related to my departure. Although I tried to broach this subject on several occasions, Ronny consistently denied being angry about my leaving.

The following week, Ronny drew pictures of events that occurred at his summer camp. He then began to draw a still-life portrait of the items I had on a bookshelf. This drawing was an exact replication of three cacti and a framed picture. Ronny told me that he would always remember this part of my office, as he always faced that part of the room during our sessions. He did not complete the picture and asked whether he could do so the following week.

Ronny chose to play Jenga instead of working on the drawing during the next session. He asked whether he could finish the picture in our last hour and requested that we have a "graduation" at that time. I asked how he would like to do that, and he said he would like to think about it. He decided to bring a present for me to our last session. It was an audiotape of nature sounds: animals, brooks, the ocean, and so forth. When I opened the present and thanked him, Ronny spontaneously told me how and why he and his mom had chosen the tape for me. He said that he knew I liked nature because of the pictures in my office and the magazines in the waiting room. This indicated that Ronny had come to see me as a separate individual with personal interests. P. Kernberg (1990) notes that this is a frequent indication of emergence from and resolution of the transference. I asked whether Ronny would like to listen to music with me, and he enthusiastically responded "Yep" and proceded to put the tape on.

During this last session Ronny worked on his still life and on a map of a museum he had visited. He also talked spontaneously about what he had seen at the museum and about how he would be graduating to a green belt in his karate class. From time to time he even demonstrated a move or two. Ronny whistled to the music while drawing. There was a zest for learning and new adventures in his voice and a clear sense of joy. After drawing his picture he asked whether we could look at other drawings he had done during our sessions. This, it turned out, was his "graduation": to walk down memory lane by means of his drawings. After reviewing his drawings (which Ronny moved through rather quickly) I asked whether he would like to take any of the pictures home with him. He chose three, a picture of a monster "that used to be in my head," a map he had drawn after a vacation, and the still-life drawing of my shelf. He spontaneously and rather affectionately announced that the picture of the shelf would remind him of me.

Ronny used the termination phase of his treatment to deal with the reality of ending, to work through separation and mourning issues, to process difficulties he had had in the past, to clarify his newly developed resources for coping, to review our work together, and, finally, to make a still-life representation of the therapy room, which was a safe "holding environment" for him. With regard to this last activity, Ronny showed the capacity to internalize the treatment through memory.

Discussion

While Ronny seemed to be back on track developmentally, I had some concerns about his relationship with his dad, his vulnerabilities with peers, and the fact that we were terminating at a time when he was nearing preadolescence. What made matters even more complicated was the hard time I had just letting go. Winnicott (1958) notes that late latency is, in fact, a "very awkward time" to end treatment: "Apart from the actual changes of puberty, there may so easily be incidents, traumatic friendships, grand passions, seductions, masturbation anxieties, which lead to exacerbations of defences or to frank anxiety" (p. 123). Winnicott suggests that it may be beneficial to see the child at relatively infrequent intervals to keep in touch. Not being able to provide this service left me with a sense of guilt at the close of Ronny's treatment. Although I realized that I had given him a positive therapeutic experience, my guilt about leaving him before a natural ending could take place kept me from seeing just how capable Ronny had become.

Fourteen months after treatment ended I heard from Ronny's mom. She told me that additional therapy had not been needed: Ronny was very happy, did excellent work in school, had a few good friends, and had a black belt in karate. His mother reported that he was not the most popular child in the class, but neither was he the most unhappy. She attributed this to the fact that Ronny now liked himself. My conversation with Mrs. J. showed how treatment continues to have an influence long after the physical goodbye. Thus it was as true for Ronny as it was for me that the ending was just a new beginning—a beginning in which he could try out, expand, revise, and fully take ownership of a new way of being in the world.

APPENDIX: STRUCTURED TECHNIQUES FOR SAYING GOODBYE

Structured activities can be useful for both planned and premature terminations. In planned situations, structured techniques can be used to involve the child in setting a date for stopping treatment that in turn, provides her or him with the opportunity to prepare for saying goodbye. With this comes the message that the child can be an active participant in the separation process. Structured activities can help the child to make the upcoming ending more tangible and to consolidate and take ownership of newfound knowledge, understanding, and skills. They can also serve to reinforce the child's accomplishments and instill a sense of pride.

Structured activities are also useful when the therapist has a limited amount of time to bring treatment to a close. This often occurs when parents and/or children decide to end treatment in an abrupt manner. In these situations, as with planned endings, structured activities can be used to:

- review what was worked on in treatment
- provide a healthy model for sharing feelings about saying goodbye
- highlight accomplishments the child has made as a result of treatment
- address issues of loss.

Having the child leave the last session with a project that she or he made gives the child something tangible to hold onto. This can help her or him remember what was learned in treatment and can serve as a metaphor and long-lasting message regarding the therapy. The more the therapist is able to reframe termination as a positive experience, wherein the child is an active participant, the more this will help the child differentiate between this significant ending and previous losses that were outside of her/his control.

ACTIVITIES TO HELP CHILDREN ANTICIPATE AND PREPARE FOR TERMINATION

A calendar (see Figure A–1) can be made with the child during the session when a termination date is set. This can be used on a weekly basis to serve as a tangible reminder of the number of remaining days until the last session. This approach is particularly helpful with young children, given their limited ability to comprehend time (Benedict and Mongoven 1996).

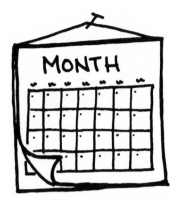

Figure A–1.   Calendar.

I have adapted this approach by using a picture of an hourglass (see Figure A–2). The hourglass is given to children at the beginning of each session and they can color in successive layers of sand in colors of their choosing. The metaphor in this activity is that the filling of the bottom half is synonymous with the child's accumulation of new skills and abilities.

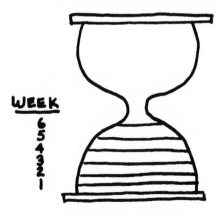

Figure A–2.   Hourglass.

Similiarly, a picture of a timeline (see Figure A–3) can be used with somewhat older children.

Figure A–3. Timeline.

ACTIVITIES TO ADDRESS LOSS ISSUES

Photographs of the play room and/or the therapist and child together are sometimes helpful for children with a history of traumatic losses (Shelby 1996). Photographing the child requires parental permission. I have adapted this technique by helping children to think of what it is about the therapy room that they would like to remember and then asking them to draw it. This provides an understanding of the child's inner experience of treatment, of what was most helpful or important to him or her, and can thus enhance communication. Some children have drawn items in the room such as a plant, picture, or piece of furniture, while others have drawn a picture of me. The activity can be used to promote the process of internalization.

Visualization is another approach for helping the child to remember and internalize the therapist. This involves instructing the child to close his or her eyes and imagine the therapist's face. When the child is able to visualize the face, the idea is conveyed that the therapist will always be retained in memory (Shelby 1996).

Hand drawings, in which the therapist's hand is outlined next to the child's (see Figure A–4), can be useful for helping the child to keep a piece of the therapist. This tangible souvenir of the partnership experienced in the therapeutic relationship can be taken out whenever the child needs to remember the therapist or requires ego support (Shelby 1996). By making two copies of the picture, one for the child and one for the therapist, the child is assured that he or she will be remembered as well.

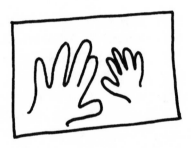

Figure A–4.   Hand drawing.

Working with the child to make a memory box (see Figure A–5) is also useful. The child gets to pick a box to decorate and fill with magazine clippings, drawings, or words depicting special lessons, feelings, coping skills, and memories in preparation for termination (Shelby 1996). Collages can be used in a similar manner.

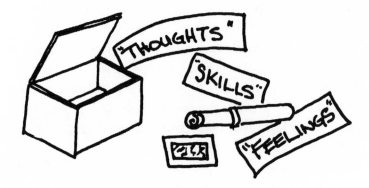

Figure A–5. Memory box.

ACTIVITIES TO CONSOLIDATE UNDERSTANDING, KNOWLEDGE, AND SKILLS

A picture of a blank coat of arms divided into four or six sections (see Figure A–6) can be used to highlight themes of the child's treatment, lessons learned, coping skills acquired, and the like. This technique can be altered depending on the age of the child and the therapeutic issues to be stressed. The approach is helpful for promoting conversation about what the child has learned in therapy. After discussing issues, the child then draws something depicting that issue or a lesson regarding it. The metaphorical message of this exercise is that the child "owns" skills and tools that are now a part of his or her identity and can be called upon whenever needed.

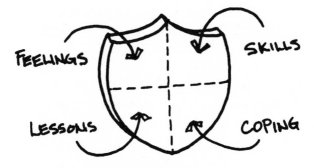

Figure A–6. Coat of arms.

A similar technique that I have called the "bag of tricks" (see Figure A–7) involves giving the child a brown paper bag to decorate. The bag is then used as a container for "tricks" or coping skills that the child has learned for dealing with feelings, problems, frustrations, likes, and dislikes. These can be depicted in magazine clippings, drawings, and/or words that are then put in the bag for the child to take home. The bag serves as a concrete reminder of the child's outer originality and internal understanding and knowledge base. Collages can be used in a similar manner.

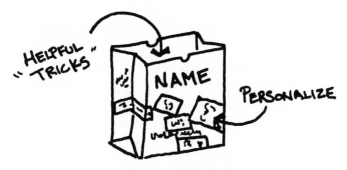

Figure A–7. Bag of tricks.

ACTIVITIES TO REINFORCE ACCOMPLISHMENTS AND INSTILL A SENSE OF PRIDE

Planting a tree (see Figure A–8) with the child can signify that termination is an accomplishment and marks a new beginning (Shelby 1996).

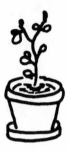

Figure A–8.   Planting a tree.

Likewise, a graduation ceremony (see Figure A–9) can be planned for the last session in order to convey a sense of accomplishment. Shelby notes that formal ceremonies may even involve having stuffed animals to participate or watch. In a more open-ended manner, the child may be told that the last session can be used as a celebration of his or her accomplishments. The child is then called upon to think of ways to celebrate, and with the help of the therapist a special event is planned. I have had children bring music, food, or special games to the session in these situations.

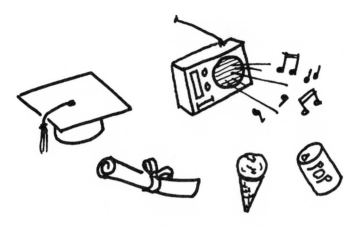

Figure A-9. Graduation ceremony.

Still another technique is for the therapist to write a short, developmentally appropriate book (see Figure A-10) about the child's history and his or her accomplishments in therapy (Benedict and Mongoven 1996). This can be read with the child, colored in by the child, and then taken home as a souvenir of the therapy experience.

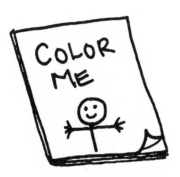

Figure A-10. Book.

REFERENCES

Allen, F. (1942). *Psychotherapy with Children*. New York: Norton.

Axline, V. (1964). *Dibs: In Search of Self*. New York: Ballantine.

Benedict, H. E., and Mongoven, L. B. (1996). Thematic play therapy: an approach to treatment of attachment disorders in young children. In *The Playing Cure*, ed. H. Kaduson, D. Cangelosi, and C. Schaefer, pp. 277–315. Northvale, NJ: Jason Aronson.

Bowlby, J. (1973). *Separation: Anxiety and Anger*. New York: Basic Books.

Cangelosi, D. (1995) *Psychodynamic Play Therapy*. In *Clinical Handbook of Anxiety Disorders in Children and Adolescents*, ed. A. R. Eisen, C. A. Kearney, and C. E. Schaefer, pp. 439–460. Northvale, NJ: Jason Aronson.

Coppolillo, H. P. (1988). *Psychodynamic Psychotherapy of Children*. Madison, CT: International Universities Press.

Deutsch, H. (1937). Absence of grief. *Psychoanalytic Quarterly* 6:12–22.

Dewald, P. A. (1980). Forced termination of psychotherapy: the annually recurrent trauma. *Psychiatric Opinion*, January, pp. 13–15.

Erikson, E. H. (1963). *Childhood and Society*. New York: Norton.

Fenster, S., Phillips, S., and Rapoport, E. (1986). *The Therapist's Pregnancy: Intrusion in the Analytic Space*. Hillsdale, NJ: Analytic Press.

Freud, A. (1962). Assessment of childhood disturbances. In *Psychoanalytic Study of the Child* 17:149–158. New York: International Universities Press.

——— (1965). *Normality and Pathology in Childhood. Assessments of Development*. Madison, CT: International Universities Press.

——— (1969). Assessment of pathology in children. In *The Writings of Anna Freud: Research at the Hampstead Child Therapy Clinic and Other Papers, Volume 5*, pp. 26–59. New York: International Universities Press.

——— (1971). Problems of termination in child analysis. In *The Writings of Anna Freud: Problems of Psychoanalytic Training, and the Technique of Therapy, Volume 7*, pp. 3–21. New York: International Universities Press.

Freud, S. (1937). *Analysis Terminable and Interminable*, ed. P. Rieff. New York: Collier.

Furman, E. (1980). Transference and externalization in latency. In *Psychoanalytic Study of the Child* 35:267–284. New Haven, CT: Yale University Press.

Furman, R. A. (1964). Death and the young child. In *Psychoanalytic Study of the Child* 19:321–333. New York: International Universities Press.

Gillman, R. D. (1991). Termination in psychotherapy with children and adolescents. In *Saying Goodbye: A Case-*

book of *Termination in Child and Adolescent Analysis and Therapy*, ed. A. G. Schmuckler, pp. 339–354. Hillsdale, NJ: Analytic Press.

Glenn, J. (1978). *Child Analysis and Therapy*. New York: Jason Aronson.

Guy, J., Guy, M., and Liaboe, G. (1986). First pregnancy: therapeutic issues for both female and male psychotherapists. *Psychotherapy* 23:297–302.

Horowitz, M., Wilner, N., Marmor, C., and Krupnick, J. (1980). Pathological grief and the activation of latent self-images. *American Journal of Psychiatry* 137(10): 1157–1162.

Johnson, J. (1996). *Toys "r" tools*. Paper presented at the second annual conference of the Colorado Association for Play Therapy. Arvada, CO, February.

Kernberg, P. F. (1991). Termination in child psychoanalysis: criteria from within the session. In *Saying Goodbye: A Casebook of Termination in Child and Adolescent Analysis and Therapy*, ed. A. G. Schmuckler, pp. 321–337. Hillsdale, NJ: Analytic Press.

Klein, M. (1932). *The Psycho-Analysis of Children*. London: Hogarth.

Levinson, H. L. (1977). Termination of psychotherapy: some salient issues. *Social Casework* 10:480–489.

Loewald, H. W. (1962). Internalization, separation, mourning and the superego. *Psychoanalytic Quarterly* 31:483–504.

——— (1988). Termination analyzable and unanalyzable. In *Psychoanalytic Study of the Child* 43:155–166. New Haven, CT: Yale University Press.

Maenchen, A. (1970). On the technique of child analysis in relation to stages of development. *Psychoanalytic Study of the Child* 25:175–208. New York: International Universities Press.

Mahler, M., Pine, F., and Bergman, A. (1975). *The Psychological Birth of the Human Infant*. New York: Basic Books.

Miller, J. R. (1992). Play therapy with young children during the pregnancy of a novice therapist. *Psychotherapy* 29:631–634.

Mozgal, A. (1985). Termination of psychotherapy: potential problems for patient and therapist. *Carrier Foundation Letter* 111, November, pp. 1–4.

Nagera, H. (1970). Children's reactions to the death of important objects. *Psychoanalytic Study of the Child* 25:360–400. New York: International Universities Press.

Novick, J., and Kelly, K. (1970). Projection and externalization. *This Annual* 25:69–95.

Parsons, M. (1990). Some issues affecting termination: the treatment of a high-risk adolescent. In *Psychoanalytic Study of the Child* 45:437–458. New Haven, CT: Yale University Press.

Pedder, J. R. (1982). Failure to mourn, and melancholia. *British Journal of Psychiatry* 141:329–337.

Piaget, J. (1951). *Play, Dreams, and Imitation in Childhood*, trans. C. Gatlegno and F. M. Hodgson. New York: Norton.

Rank, O. (1929). *The Trauma of Birth*. New York: Brunner, 1952.

Robinson, H. (1991). Visitation with divorced father provokes reemergence of unresolved family conflicts: case of Charlie, age 10. In *Play Therapy with Children in Crisis*, ed. N. Boyd-Webb, pp. 217–236. New York: Guilford.

Sandler, J., Kennedy, H., and Tyson, R. L. (1980). *The Technique of Child Psychoanalysis: Discussions with Anna Freud*. Cambridge, MA: Harvard University Press.

Schaefer, C. (1996). *Words of Wisdom for Parents: Time-*

Tested Thoughts on How to Raise Kids. Northvale, NJ: Jason Aronson.

Schechter, M. D., and Combrinck-Graham, L. (1980). The normal development of the seven-to-ten-year-old child. In *The Course of Life: Psychoanalytic Contributions Toward Understanding Personality Development. Vol. 2: Latency, Adolescence, and Youth*, ed. S. I. Greenspan and G. H. Pollock, pp. 83–107. Adelphi, MD: Mental Health Study Center, National Institute of Mental Health.

Sekaer, C., and Katz, S. (1986). On the concept of mourning in childhood. In *Psychoanalytic Study of the Child* 41:287–314. New Haven, CT: Yale University Press.

Shelby, J. (1996). *Post-traumatic play therapy for survivors of acute abuse and community violence*. Paper presented at the eleventh annual Summer Play Therapy seminars, Hackensack, NJ, July.

Shulman, T. (1996). Personal communication, July.

Solnit, A. J. (1987). A psychoanalytic view of play. In *Psychoanalytic Study of the Child* 42:205–219. New Haven, CT: Yale University Press.

Spiegel, S. (1989). *An Interpersonal Approach to Child Therapy: The Treatment of Children and Adolescents from an Interpersonal Point of View*. New York: Columbia University Press.

Van Dam, H., Heinicke, C. M., and Shane, M. (1975). On termination in child analysis. In *Psychoanalytic Study of the Child* 30:443–474. New Haven, CT: Yale University Press.

Viorst, J. (1986). *Necessary Losses*. New York: Fawcett Gold Medal.

Weiss, S. (1991). Vicissitudes of termination: transferences and countertransferences. In *Saying Goodbye: A Casebook of Termination in Child and Adolescent Analysis and Therapy*, ed. A. G. Schmuckler, pp. 265–284. Hillsdale, NJ: Analytic Press.

Winnicott, D. W. (1958). Child analysis in the latency period. In *The Maturational Process and the Facilitative Environment*. New York: International Universities Press.

———— (1963). From dependence towards independence in the development of the individual. In *The Maturational Process and the Facilitative Environment*. New York: International Universities Press.

Wolfenstein, M. (1966). How is mourning possible? In *Psychoanalytic Study of the Child* 21:93–121. New York: International Universities Press.

———— (1969). Loss, rage, and repetition. In *Psychoanalytic Study of the Child* 24:432–460. New York: International Universities Press.

INDEX

ABOUT THE AUTHOR

Donna Cangelosi, Psy.D., is an instructor in child and adolescent psychotherapy at the New Jersey Institute for Psychoanalysis in Teaneck, New Jersey. She is a member of the Association for Play Therapy and the American Psychological Association. Co-editor of the books *Play Therapy Techniques* and *The Playing Cure*, she has authored several chapters on psychodynamic treatment with children. Dr. Cangelosi has lectured throughout the country on topics related to separation, loss, and divorce issues in children; psychodynamic play therapy; and the ending phase of treatment. She maintains a private psychotherapy practice with children, adolescents, and adults in Teaneck.